Advances in Anatomy, Embryology and Cell Biology
Ergebnisse der Anatomie und Entwicklungsgeschichte
Revues d'anatomie et de morphologie expérimentale

52/2

W0043100

Editors

A. Brodal, Oslo · W. Hild, Galveston · J. van Limborgh, Amsterdam
R. Ortmann, Köln · T. H. Schiebler, Würzburg · G. Töndury, Zürich · E. Wolff, Paris

Pierre Cau, Marc Michel-Béchet, Guy Fayet

Morphogenesis
of Thyroid Follicles in Vitro

With 16 Figures

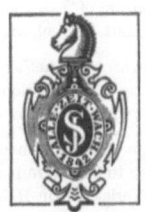

Springer-Verlag Berlin Heidelberg New York 1976

Pierre Cau, Marc Michel-Béchet, Guy Fayet
Laboratoire d'Histologie I
Faculté de Médecine
F-13385 Marseille Cedex 4
France

This work was supported by CNRS and INSERM (Unit 38)

ISBN-13:978-3-540-07654-4   e-ISBN-13:978-3-642-66334-5
DOI: 10.1007/978-3-642-66334-5

Library of Congress Cataloging in Publication Data. Cau, P. 1947 — Morphogenesis of thyroid follicles in vitro. (Advances in anatomy, embryology, and cell biology; v. 52, fasc. 2). Includes bibliographical references and index. 1. Thyroid gland. 2. Morphogenesis. 3. Organs, Culture of. I. Michel-Béchet, M., 1929 — joint author. II. Fayet, G., 1940 — joint author. III. Title. IV. Series. QL801.E67 vol. 52, fasc. 2 [QL868]574.4'08s[591.1'42]76—7969

Contents

Introduction

The thyroid gland first appears in the phylogenic scale in the Lamprey larva, Ammocoetes, at the time of metamorphosis (see review by Constantinescu, 1972). In higher Vertebrates the adult thyroid gland consists of vesicles i. e. thyroid follicles containing colloid and lined with a cubic or prismatic epithelium.

Since the end of the 19th century, many authors have studied the morphogenesis of the follicles during the embryonic and fetal development of the gland in Man and other species, principally Chick, Rat and Rabbit.

The development of techniques for culturing organs of higher animals, in particular the thyroid by Carrel and Burrows (1910) and Champy (1914, 1915), allowed the study of the survival *in vivo* or *in vitro* of grafts or explants of thyroid gland obtained from adult or fetal animals. In addition to organotypic cultures, techniques for culturing cell suspensions obtained by enzymatic dissociation have recently been refined.

Moreover, histological examination of pathological human glands and adult thyroids experimentally stimulated by thyrotropin hormone (TSH) has provided additional data for the understanding of thyroid follicle morphogenesis.

Since the earliest work, two opposing hypotheses have been put forward to explain the mechanism of follicular formation. According to the first hypothesis, the fetal thyroid is a tubular gland in the pre-follicular stage, either because the thyroid primordium is itself hollow right from its appearance at the pharyngeal floor, or because a channel appears in the thyroid primordium after the separation of this structure from the entoblastic epithelium. The thyroid follicles are formed by constriction of the glandular tube, or by segmentation of this tube by connective tissue and blood vessels which invade the primordium. The adult thyroid gland partially or totally keeps the embryonic tubular structure next to the newly built, follicular architecture. These phenomena have been described in Man (Muller, 1971; Kölliker, 1884; Streiff, 1897; Hertwig, 1906; Prenant et al,. 1911; Simpson, 1912; Biedl, 1913; Weil, 1922; Hammar, 1925; Cooper, 1925; Pulaski, 1929; Stefko, 1934; Loeschke, 1937), in the Rat (Florentin, 1932), in the Rabbit (Kölliker, 1884), in the Chick (Remak, 1885) and teleostean Fishes (Florentin, 1932).

In the second hypothesis, the adult thyroid gland is composed of a great number of juxtaposed follicles sometimes interjoined by epithelial cords devoid of a lumen. The early embryonic thyroid is first formed by solid cell cords. Budding, constriction or invasion by connective strands and vessels result in fragmentation of these epithelial cords into small cell clumps which are most often solid. The thyroid follicles originate from these isolated clumps and the follicular lumen then appears after radial rearrangement of the epithelial cells in the following three different ways:

first, the lumen arises from necrosis or liquefaction of the cells situated in the center of the cell clump or from lysis of the cellular centripetal pole, by a mechanism analogous to that of apocrine secretion. This is the case in Man according to Peremeschko (1867); Wölfler, (1883); Stieda (1881); His (1885); Langendorff (1889); Lucien et al. (1925) and in the Pig according to Lustig (1891);

second, the lumen appears between the cells, then grows larger by secretion of colloid or a precursor of colloid into the intercellular space or center of the cell clump (Fig. 1a). Proposed after the early works on embryonic thyroid in Man (Marshall, 1893; Tourneux and Verdun, 1897; Grosser, 1912; Gierke, 1913; Norris, 1916; Bucciante and Maspes, 1930; Takashima and Hara, 1934; Bargmann, 1956; Sugiyama, 1971; Lietz et al., 1971), in the Rat (Sugiyama, 1941; Hall and Kaan, 1942; Chardard-Raimbault, 1953; Carpenter and Rondon-Tarchetti, 1958; Feldman et al., 1961; Ishikawa, 1965), in the Rabbit (Florentin, 1932; Togari et al., 1952; Roques et al., 1973), in the Ox (Eguchi and Hashimoto, 1959), in the Chick (Bonnet, 1891; Hopkins, 1935; Stoll et al., 1953; Maraud and Stoll, 1961; Hajos et al., 1964; Hilfer, 1964; Fujita and Tanizawa, 1966), in Amphibians (Schrecken-berg, 1956; Nonaka, 1956; Nonaka et al., 1959), in some Fish (Hoar, 1939), this process of thyroid follicle formation from the space separating the epithelial cells from each other was also observed in the Lamprey larva at the time of appearance of the thyroid gland (Kraentzel, 1933; Leach, 1939; Clements-Merlini, 1960; Con-stantinescu, 1972; Suzuki and Kondo, 1973), in embryonic Chick thyroid cultures (Sobel and Leurer, 1958; Petrovic and Porte, 1961; Daems and Thesing, 1962; Hilfer et al., 1968; Spooner, 1970), in thyroid cultures from adult Rat (Junqueira, 1947) and Pig (Michel-Béchet et al., 1973) and finally at the time of vesicular differen-tiation of the interfollicular epithelial cell clumps in the Dog (Hurthle, 1894);

third, each cell in the clump becomes hollow by formation of an intracyto-plasmic cavity considered to be an elementary microfollicle. The mature follicular lumen arises from the more or less simultaneous fusion of neighbouring cells cavities (Fig. 1b). This mechanism has been favoured by authors studying the embryonic thyroid of Man (Horcika, 1880; Shepard, 1968; Garcia-Bunuel et al., 1972), Rat (Van Heyningen, 1961; Voikevitch and Zenzerov, 1968; Welsch, 1972; Calvert and Pusterla, 1973), Ox (Koneff et al., 1949), Chick (Bradway, 1929; Venzke, 1949; Macario, 1954; Kraicziczek, 1956; Fujita and Machino, 1961). In addition cultures of human (Shepard, 1967) and Chick (Gaillard, 1953; Kojima, 1960) embryonic thyroids, cultures of Rat (Junqueira, 1947) and Rabbit (Knake and Riedel, 1960) adult glands and TSH-stimulated cultures of adult Dog thyroid (Neve and Dumont, 1970) lead to the same conclusion. Finally, certain follicles of human pathological glands could be formed in this way especially in toxic nodule (Michel-Béchet et al., 1968) and in goitres (Heiman, 1966).

Evidence acquired due to progressive improvement of light microscopy tech-niques and by use of the electron microscope has allowed the first hypothesis to be discarded. The adult thyroid gland is not partially or totally tubular nor does the early thyroid at the stage of folliculogenesis have a tubular structure.

In the second place, modern histological techniques have not been able to demonstrate central necrosis of the solid cell clump nor phenomena of apocrine secretion responsible for the appearance of the follicular lumen according to the second hypothesis.

Only two different mechanisms for the formation of the follicular lumen inside the solid cell clumps composing the primordium are currently considered, namely the secretion of colloid or a precursor by the thyroid cells into the space between them, and the simultaneous fusion of intracytoplasmic microfollicular colloid-containing cavities which appear individually in adjacent cells.

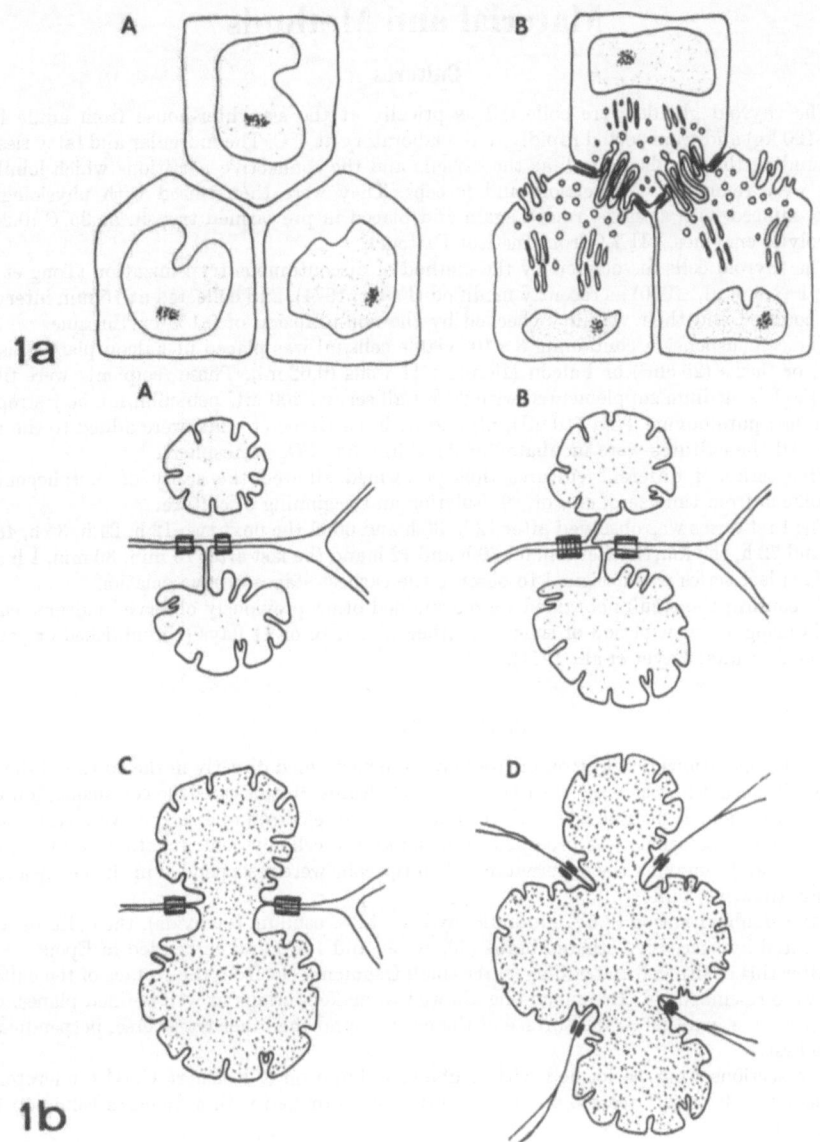

Fig. 1 (a). Formation of the follicular lumen from the intercellular space, after Hilfer, (b) Formation of the follicular lumen by simultaneous fusion of originally intracytoplasmic cavities, after Shepard

Since one of us had already studied some aspects of follicular morphogenesis *in vivo*, and another had developed a method of cell culture *in vitro* adapted to thyroid cells, we wanted to take advantage of this to investigate this problem using *in vitro* cultures of trypsin-dissociated thyroid cells in the broader frame of the epithelial cells sociology and interactions[1].

1 This work is a continuation of previous investigation by Prof. M. Michel-Béchet and Dr. G. Fayet, and its results have been related in a thesis for the Doctorate of Medicine by P. Cau

Material and Methods

Cultures

The thyroid glands were collected aseptically at the slaughter-house from adult Pigs (100–120 kg) and transported rapidly to the laboratory at 4°C. The muscular and fatty tissues surrounding the glands, as well as the capsule and the connective partitions which lobulate them were removed with scissors and forceps. They were then rinsed with physiological saline, minced with scissors, rinsed again and placed in prewarmed trypsin at 35°C (0.25% proteolytic enzymes, pH 7.0 from Institut Pasteur).

The thyroid cells dissociated by the method of discontinuous trypsinization (Tong et al., 1962; Fayet et al., 1970) as recently modified (Fayet, 1974), and collected at 15 min intervals were counted and their viability checked by the non-diffusion of 0.1% erythrosine.

The cell suspension containing 3×10^6 viable cells/ml was placed in Falcon plastic dishes (2 ml) or flasks (25 cm²) or Falcon Microtest II wells (0.02 ml). These recipients were filled with Eagle's medium supplemented with 20% Calf serum, 200 mU penicillin/ml, 50 γ streptomycin/ml; pure bovine TSH (40 mU/ml) and hydrocortisone (1 γ/ml) were added to the medium. All the cultures were incubated at 35°C in a 5% CO_2 atmosphere.

Five series of different cultures thus performed allowed the study of morphogenetic phenomena from time zero, end of cell isolation and beginning of culture.

The first series was observed after 12 h, 36 h and 60 h, the next two 12 h, 24 h, 36 h, 48 h, 60 h and 72 h, the fourth after 3 h, 6 h, 9 h and 12 h and the last after 15 min, 30 min, 1 h and 3 h. This last series was designed to observe the earliest stages of reassociation.

To confirm the results obtained we reexamined other previously observed cultures cultivated during a longer period of time i. e. either 4, 6, 7, 10 or 11 days (Unpublished or partly published results: Fayet et al., 1971).

Electron Microscopy

All the operations for electron microscopy were performed directly in the culture dishes or microwells except for the very short-time (0–3 h) cultures. In this case, the cell suspension was tipped into a hemolysis tube where all the operations for electron microscopy were performed. Each of these operations was preceded by pelleting the cells by centrifugation at 1,000 rpm for 10 min and removing the supernatant; then the cells were resuspended in the newly added medium (fixative, buffer,...).

After double fixation (2.5% glutaraldehyde and 2% osmium tetroxide), the cultures were dehydrated by successive ethanol baths (50, 70, 90 and 100°) and embedded in Epon.

After this in situ cell embedding, three small fragments cut from the surface of the culture flask were re-embedded. Re-embedding allowed to make sections in well defined planes, one tangential, i. e. parallel to the surface of the culture, and the other transverse, perpendicular to the first.

The sections were performed with a diamond knife on a Reichert OMU 1 microtome, contrasted with uranyl acetate and lead citrate and examined with a Siemens Elmiscop 101 microscope.

In addition, serial sections were obtained from cultures treated with TSH during 3 h and 12 h respect. In the tangential section, 14 grids each supporting an average of 10 sections about 800 Å thick were collected. The whole thickness of the culture, namely 10 μ, was thus explored. In the transverse plane the same method was used to explore a similar length.

Results

I. Freshly Dissociated Cells

At the onset of culture the ultrastructural appearance of the pig thyroid cells is the same as that of cells isolated from the thyroids of Man (Shimazaki et al., 1967), Sheep (Neve et al., 1968; Tixier-Vidal et al., 1969), Chick (Hilfer & Hilfer, 1966). The cell pellet contains many totally isolated elements but also follicle fragments comprising 2–10 epithelial cells always interjoined at their apical pole. It also contains cell debris resulting from trypsinization, a few red cells and some connective elements such as mastocytes, macrophages and lymphocytes.

A. The Isolated Cells

The isolated cells are spherical and measure about 8 μ in diameter (Fig. 2). The polarity characteristic of thyroid epithelium *in vivo* has completely disappeared.

The plasma membrane is devoid of apical microvilli as well as of cytoplasmic protrusions normally found on the lateral faces (Young, 1966). In addition, the plasma membrane seems inert and shows no activity related to endocytosis or exocytosis. Junctional complex joining *in vivo* thyroid cells together by their apical pole has often totally disappeared. Sometimes a small zone of membrane densification persists which some authors (Overton, 1962, 1968; Overton and Culver, 1973; Borysenko and Revel, 1973) have interpreted as being half of a desmosome. A more or less complete junctional complex can occasionally be seen between two cells, one intact and the other destroyed, the latter only recognizable by the ghost of its plasma membrane.

The round but often notched nucleus measures 3 μ in diameter. The chromatin is most frequently condensed in large clumps along the nuclear membrane.

The cytoplasmic organelles are those of a thyroid cell. The Golgi apparatus is often visible and extends around the nucleus. The small-sized mitochondria are in close contact with the endoplasmic reticulum (E. R.) cisternae. These cisternae, sometimes distended, bear an array of ribosomes analogous to that seen *in vivo* and contain a very poorly contrasted material. A great number of dense bodies of variable size (0.1–1 μ) and irregular shape, surrounded by a single membrane, are also noted.

B. The Fragments of the Follicle Epithelium

The fragments of the follicle epithelium have an appearance very similar to that of the gland *in vivo* (Fig. 3). The cells frequently keep a well defined polarity marked by the presence of several apical microvilli and the position of the nucleus at the opposite pole. The lateral surfaces are occasionally provided with numerous cytoplasmic extensions which are branched an entangled with those of neighbouring cells. The organelles do not show any modifications related to cells being isolated; only the abundance of large dense bodies is striking.

The cells are joined by a typical junctional complex associating a zonula occludens, a desmosome and occasionally a zonula adherens (Fig. 3d). At the extremity of the follicle fragment, the same localized membrane densification as has been described in the totally isolated cells can be encountered.

At this time of culture no difference exists between the TSH-stimulated and non-stimulated cells.

II. Unreassociated Cells

The thyroid cells which do not show an image of re-association are those which are still isolated after 15 min or those observed after 4 days in culture.

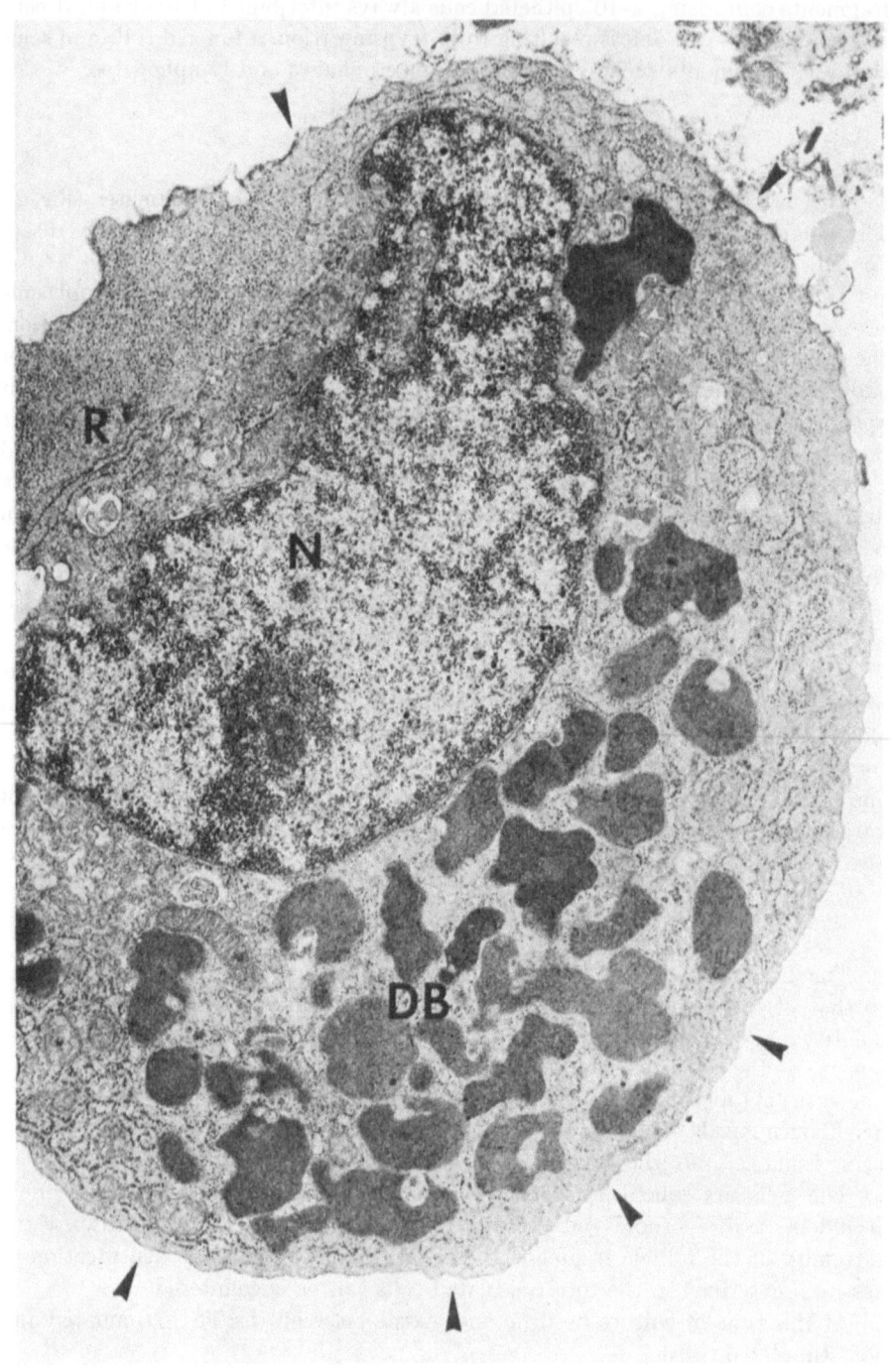

Fig. 2. Isolated TSH-stimulated cell after 15 min culture. Absence of peripheral cytoplasmic extensions (▶); notched nucleus (N); numerous dense bodies (DB); numerous free ribosomes (R). ×16,500

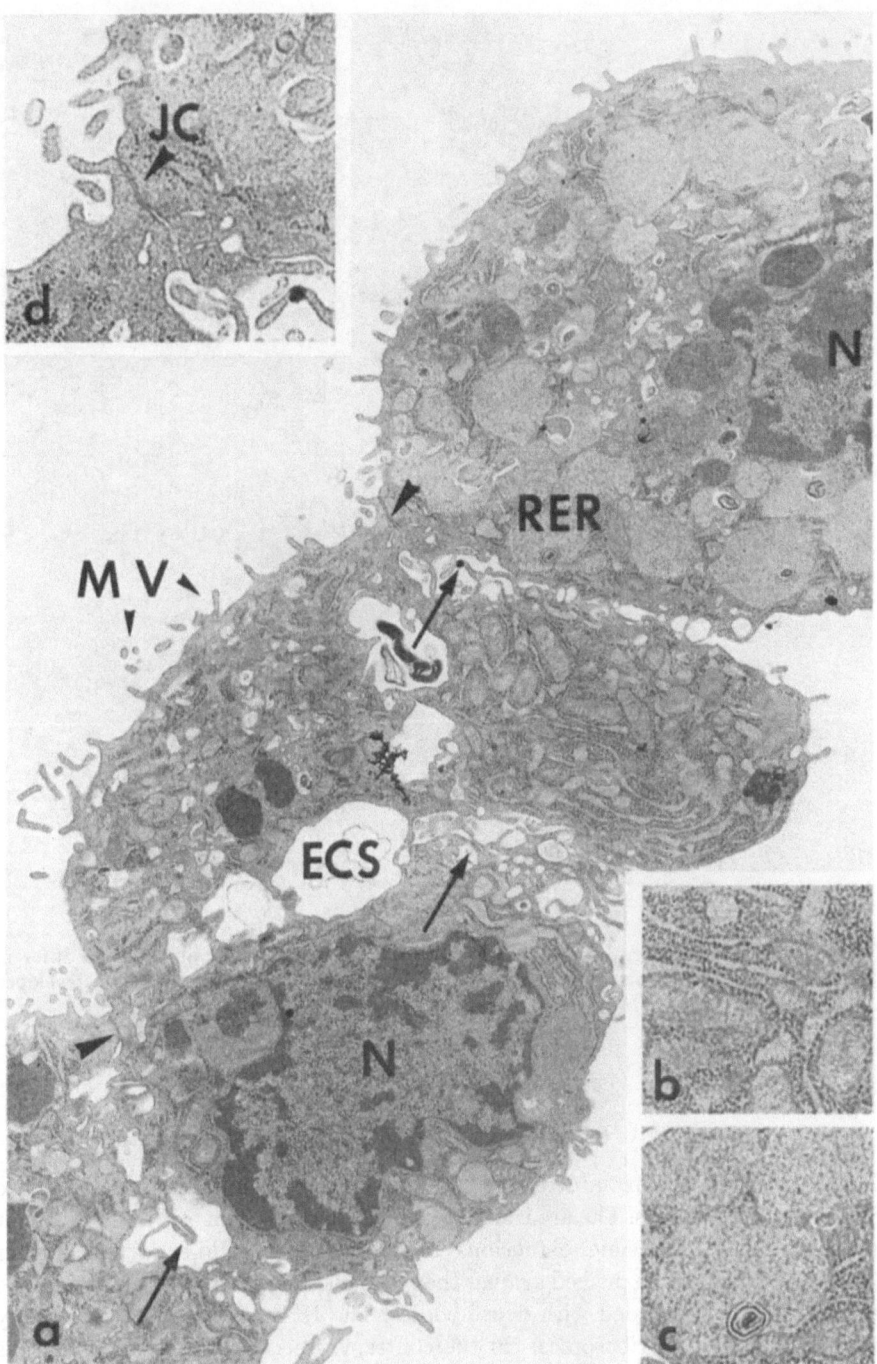

Fig. 3a—d. Fragment of incompletely dissociated follicular epithelium after 15 min culture in the absence of TSH. (a) General view; conservation of the polarity with microvilli (*MV*) and apical cell junctions (▶); notched nucleus (*N*); distended lateral cell spaces (*ECS*) with finger-like cytoplasmic extensions (→). ×12,000. (b) and (c) Two aspects of the endoplasmic reticulum (*RE*) in two adjacent cells. (d) Apical junctional complex (*JC*) that had resisted enzymatic hydrolysis. b, c, d: ×24,000

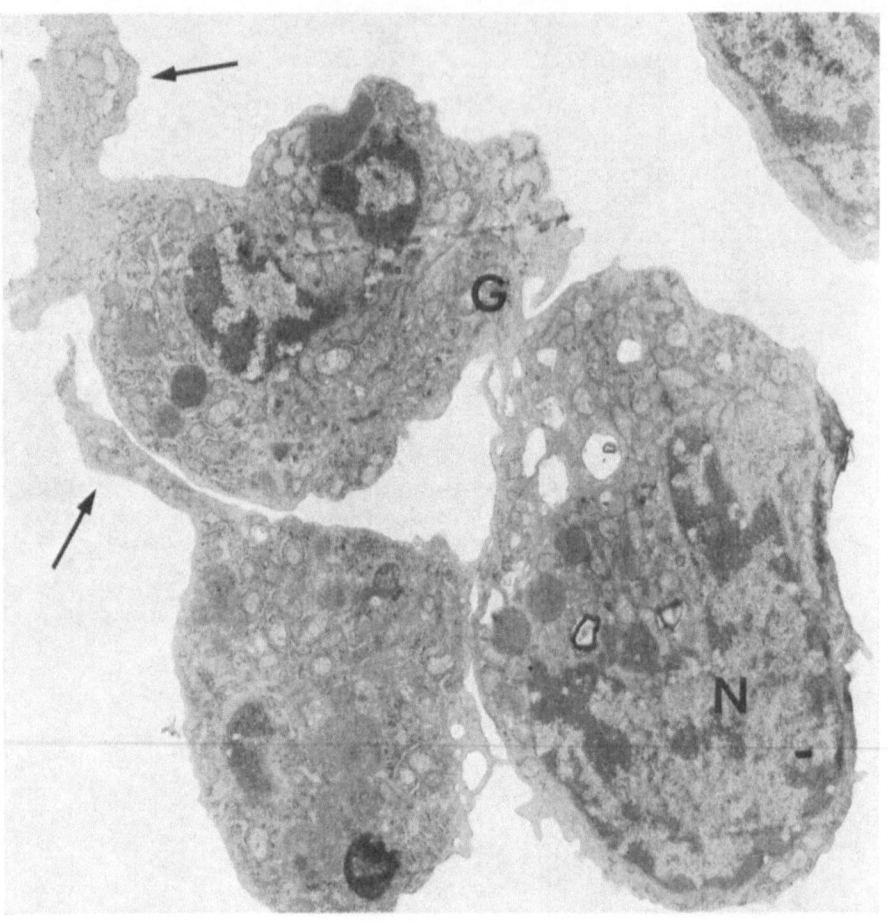

Fig. 4. Control culture after 3 h. Small aggregate of three thyroid cells; absence of a differentiated cell junction; voluminous cytoplasmic extensions (→); notched nucleus (N); developed
Golgi apparatus (G). ×11,000

A. Control Cells after 15 min Culture

The control cells examined after 15 min culture have a similar aspect to
freshly trypsinized cells. The are isolated, keep a rounded form and do not present
microvilli nor cytoplasmic extensions nor vesicles of endo-exocytosis. Their
notched nucleus is often pushed against the plasmalemma by the extreme widening
of the Golgi area, crowded with dense bodies. The E. R. cisternae have partially
lost their covering of ribosomes. On the contrary, free ribosomes are numerous
in the hyaloplasma.

The fragments of follicle epithelium are still present, but the cells of which
they are composed have become very similar to isolated cells. They have lost
their microvilli and their lateral and basal cytoplasmic extensions, but they
remain joined at their apical pole by a junctional complex which appears highly
developed.

After 15 min culture the first manifestations of reassociation are observed between the cells still in suspension in the medium and, at the same time, between the cells already attached to the surface of the Falcon flask. However, the dissociated cells are still numerous and form clumps on the plastic support, but no cell junctions are found within these clumps (Fig. 4).

Their plasmalemma is no longer inert as before. Small cytoplasmic extensions, different from microvilli, start to rise out of the cell surface while numerous vesicles containing a clear substance, probably from endocytosis, are seen in the peripheral cytoplasm. The cells spread over the plastic support stretching out rather bulky pseudopodia which contain more or less distended cisternae the membranes of which are provided with few ribosomes, although there are numerous ribosomes in the hyaloplasma. Only the membranes of the endoplasmic reticulum remaining in close contact with mitochondria keep on a small surface their normal granular cover.

These reticular cisternae often take on a circular shape forming targetlike figures bearing two or more concentric cavities. The centre of these figures contains a finely granular electron-dense material comparable to the content of some dense bodies. These aspects emphasize the autophagic phenomena which occur in these cells. The well-developed Golgi apparatus keeps a high activity evidenced by the budding of numerous, often coated vesicles. Thick bundles of microfilaments become visible in the peripheral cytoplasm and in the vicinity of the Golgi region.

B. Control Cells after 4 or More Days in Culture

After 4 days in culture nothing resembling a follicle can still be seen if the cells have not been stimulated by TSH. The previously existing follicles seem to open and release their content into the extra-cellular medium. The culture consists of large clumps comprising 20 or more cells joined together by small desmosomes. The few small-sized microvilli persist only on the surface of the cells bordering the clump. Then all the cells lose their polarity, their organelles undergo a second functional involution. The Golgi area is reduced, the E. R. cisternae break up into a small number of short channels. After one week a characteristic monolayer culture is established (Fayet et al., 1971).

III. The Reassociated Cells

The first signs of follicular re-association are observed 15 min after stimulation of the cells by TSH. However, the same phenomenon seems to occur after the same lapse of time in the control cultures (without TSH).

A. Small Aggregates

Small clumps are formed in the culture either attached or unattached to the surface of the plastic dish (Fig. 4). The cells in these clumps have no differentiated cell junctions and show no polarity.

B. The Early Follicle

The early follicular lumen consists of a narrow cleft between two epithelial cells about 6 μ long and 0.5 μ wide (Figs. 5a, b, 6a, b).

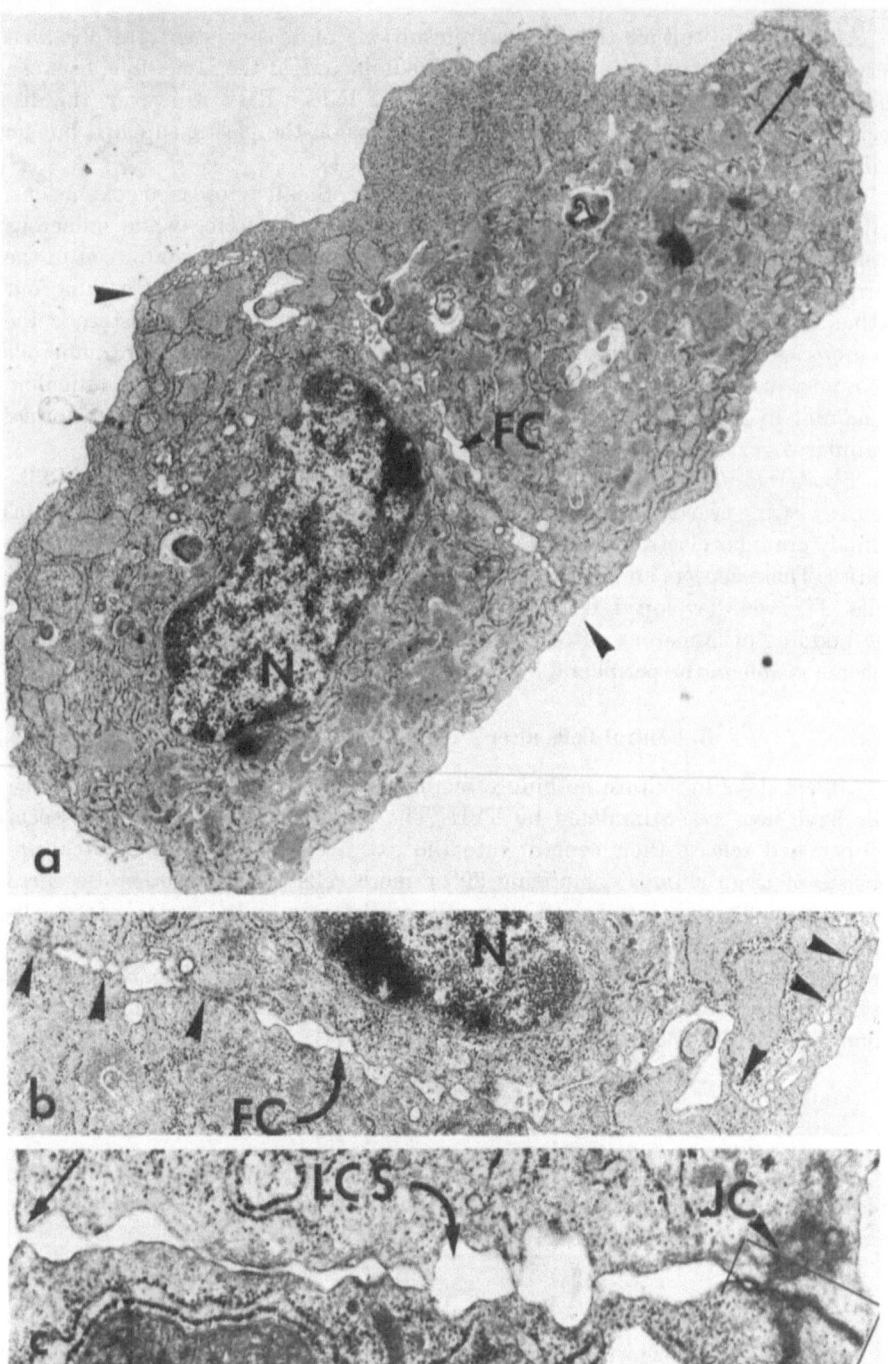

Fig. 5a—c. TSH-stimulated culture, 15 min. (a) Formation of the follicular cleft (*FC*) between two adjoining cell (▶); adult junctional complex(→) proving that one of these cells belongs to a fragment of incompletely dissociated follicular epithelium. Nucleus (*N*). ×11,000. (b) Enlargement of the follicular cleft (*FC*); numerous points of contact between the two cells (▶) constituting a primordial zonula occludens. Nucleus (*N*). ×17,500. (c) Lateral cell space (*LCS*) between two cells belonging to a fragment of incompletely dissociated thyroid epithelium; absence of cell junction at one of the two extremities of this space (→); compare the adult junctional complex (*JC*) with the cell contacts in the preceding figure. ×24,000

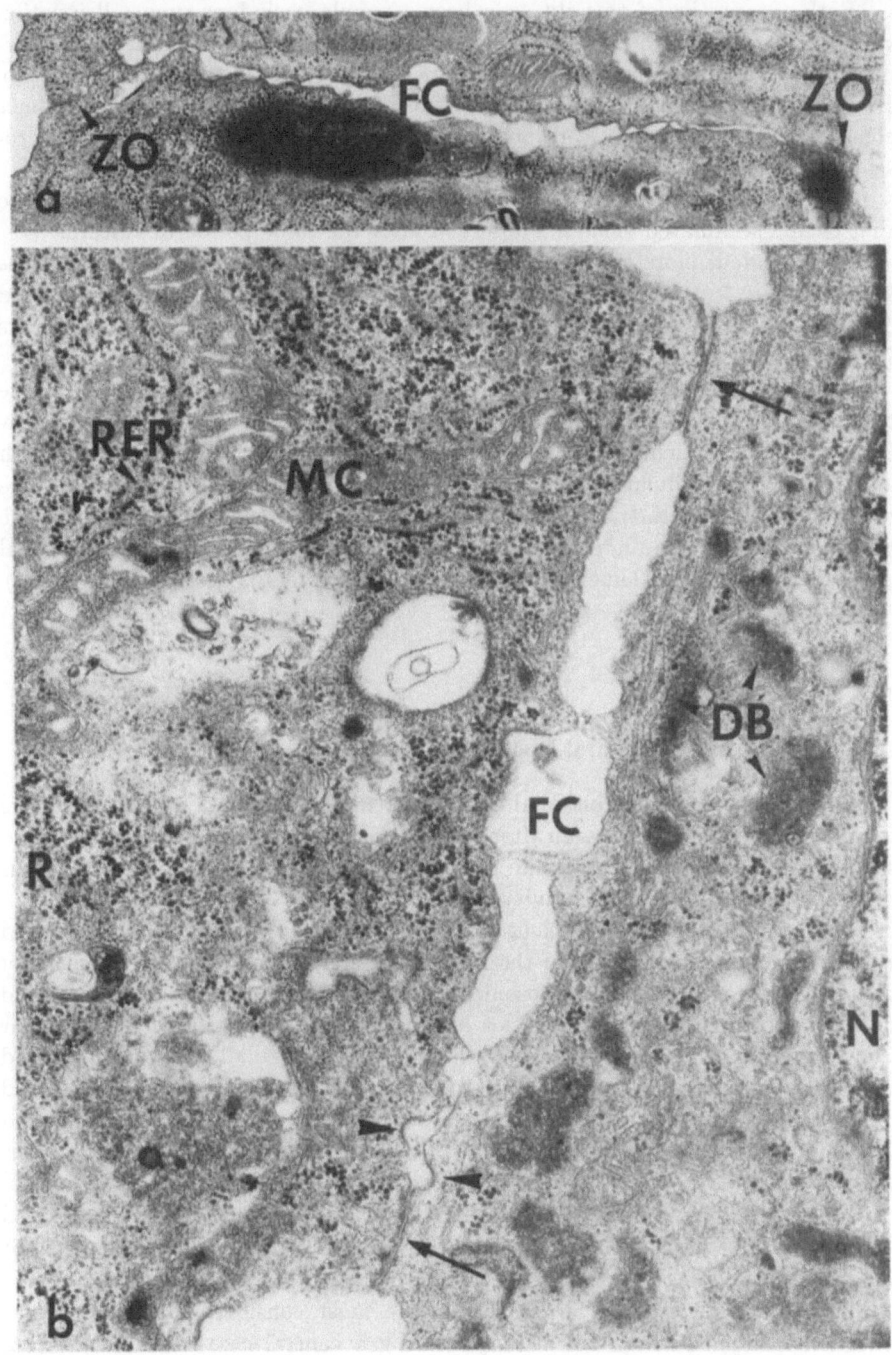

Fig. 6(a). TSH-stimulated culture, 15 min. Follicular cleft (*FC*) bounded by an annular zonula occludens (*ZO*). ×12,000. (b) Control culture in the presence of hydrocortisone, 60 h. Follicular cleft (*FC*) identical to that in Fig. 6a; zonula occludens (→); "coated" endocytotic vesicles (▶); mitochondria (*MC*); endoplasmic reticulum (*RER*); dense bodies (*DB*); free ribosomes (*R*); nucleus (*N*). ×35,000

Both extremities of this slit soon bear a zonula occludens-type cell junction which extends for about 0.5 μ. This cell junction is never associated with a desmosome or a zonula adherens, which occurs on the other hand in the adult follicle. Between these two limits the plasma membranes face each other and sometimes come in contact though no cell junction can be detected with the electron microscope. This follicular lumen appears completely empty.

The cytoplasmic ultrastructure of these re-associated cells is comparable to that of non-stimulated elements observed after the same period of culture.

The rounded, more or less central nucleus is surrounded by numerous dense bodies and by an annular cytoplasmic area where partially degranulated and often dilated E. R. cisternae are found close to several mitochondria and numerous free ribosomes.

No cell polarity is detectable at this stage of re-association and it is impossible to state with certainty that the narrow intercellular space will give rise a few hours later to a follicular cavity. Nevertheless, this cleft cannot be confused with an ordinary intercellular space as is seen in follicle fragments wherein cells have not all been separated. In this latter case a zonula occludens is never found at the basal pole of the cells and, in addition, at the apical pole there is an adult junctional complex with its three elements, but never an isolated zonula occludens (Fig. 5 b,c).

C. Ultrastructural Modifications of the Reassociated Cells

Re-association of the epithelial cells brings about considerable morphological modifications which can be seen after 3 h culture in the presence of TSH. A characteristic new polarity appears while the cytoplasmic organelles show all the signs of an increase in functional activity (Figs. 7 a, 8, 9).

The often nucleolated nucleus and the numerous dense bodies described before are displaced away from the follicular cleft by the great development of the Golgi region. Several dictyosomes line up along the follicular lumen, and numerous, sometimes coated vesicles bud off from distended saccules and near the new apical membrane. The Golgi zone contains small, irregularly-shaped vesicles containing an osmiophilic material. Numerous microfilaments and microtubules are seen in the cytoplasm, especially between the follicle lumen and the Golgi apparatus. Free ribosomes are still scattered in the hyaloplasm. However, regranulation of E. R. cisternae appears frequently in the vicinity of the mitochondria, which are less often isolated in the hyaloplasm than closely associated with the E. R. In addition, inclusions, probably of a lipidic nature, appear at the basal pole of the cells after 12 h culture.

The plasma membrane is the site of the most considerable modifications. Short intermingled microvilli already bearing a central core of microfilaments appear in the follicular lumen which is completely filled with a very dense material. Several small desmosomes form beyond, but close to the zonula occludens. Cytoplasmic extensions, longer and thinner than the microvilli and devoid of microfilaments, extend over the whole cell surface with the exception of the apical pole. Finally, numerous clear endocytotic vesicles, sometimes large in size, are visible in the peripheral cytoplasm.

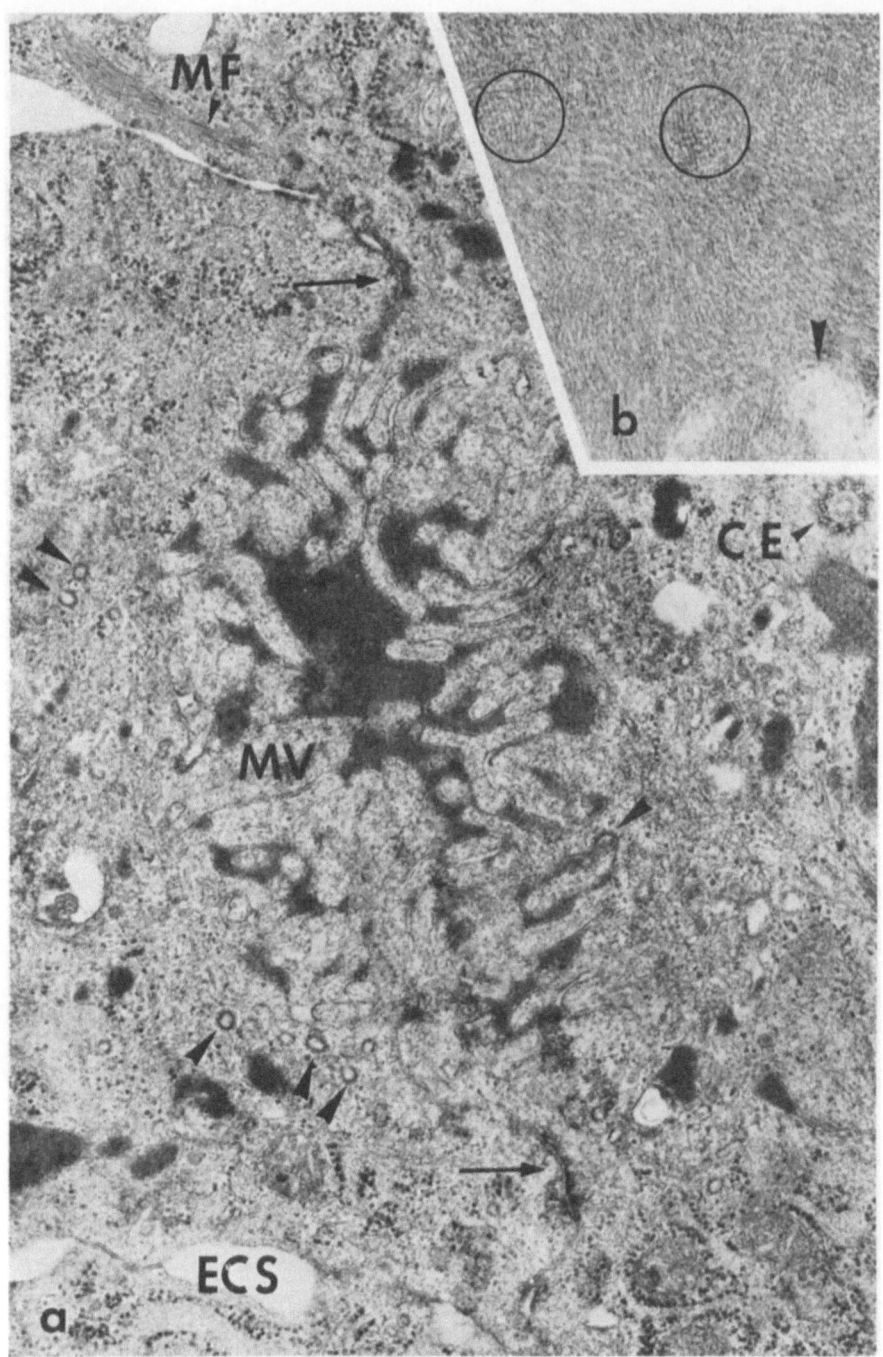

Fig. 7a a. b. TSH-stimulated culture in the presence of hydrocortisone, 12 h. (a) numerous microvilli (*MV*) and dense material filling the follicular lumen which is delimited by two sections (→) of the junctional complex; numerous "coated" vesicles (▶) originating from the follicular lumen or the Golgi apparatus; bundle of microfilaments (*MF*); centriole (*CE*); intercellular space (*ECS*). ×35,000. (b) Enlargement of the dense follicular material; in contact with the microvilli (▶), aspect of orientated filaments or tubules (circle) depending on the plane of section. ×80,000

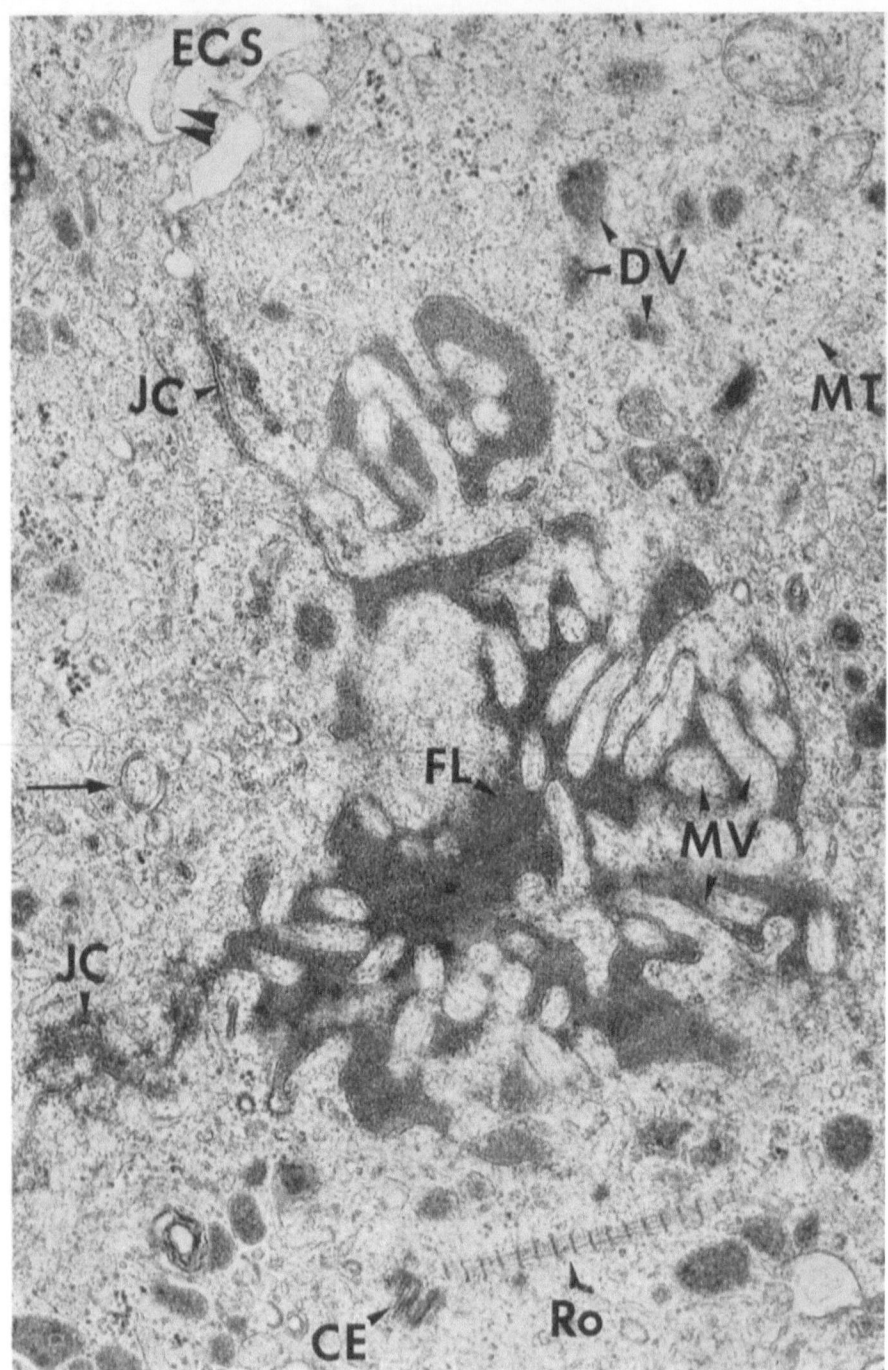

Fig. 8. TSH-stimulated culture in the presence of hydrocortisone, 12 h. Microvilli (*MV*) and dense material occupying the follicular lumen (*FL*), which is delimited by a junctional complex (*JC*); centriole (*CE*), ciliary rootlet (*Ro*) in the vicinity of the lumen; vesicles (*DV*) containing dense material; double-walled vesicle (→). Compare the difference in size of the microvilli (*MV*) and the cytoplasmic extensions (◄) in the intercellular spaces; microtubules (*MT*). ×25,000

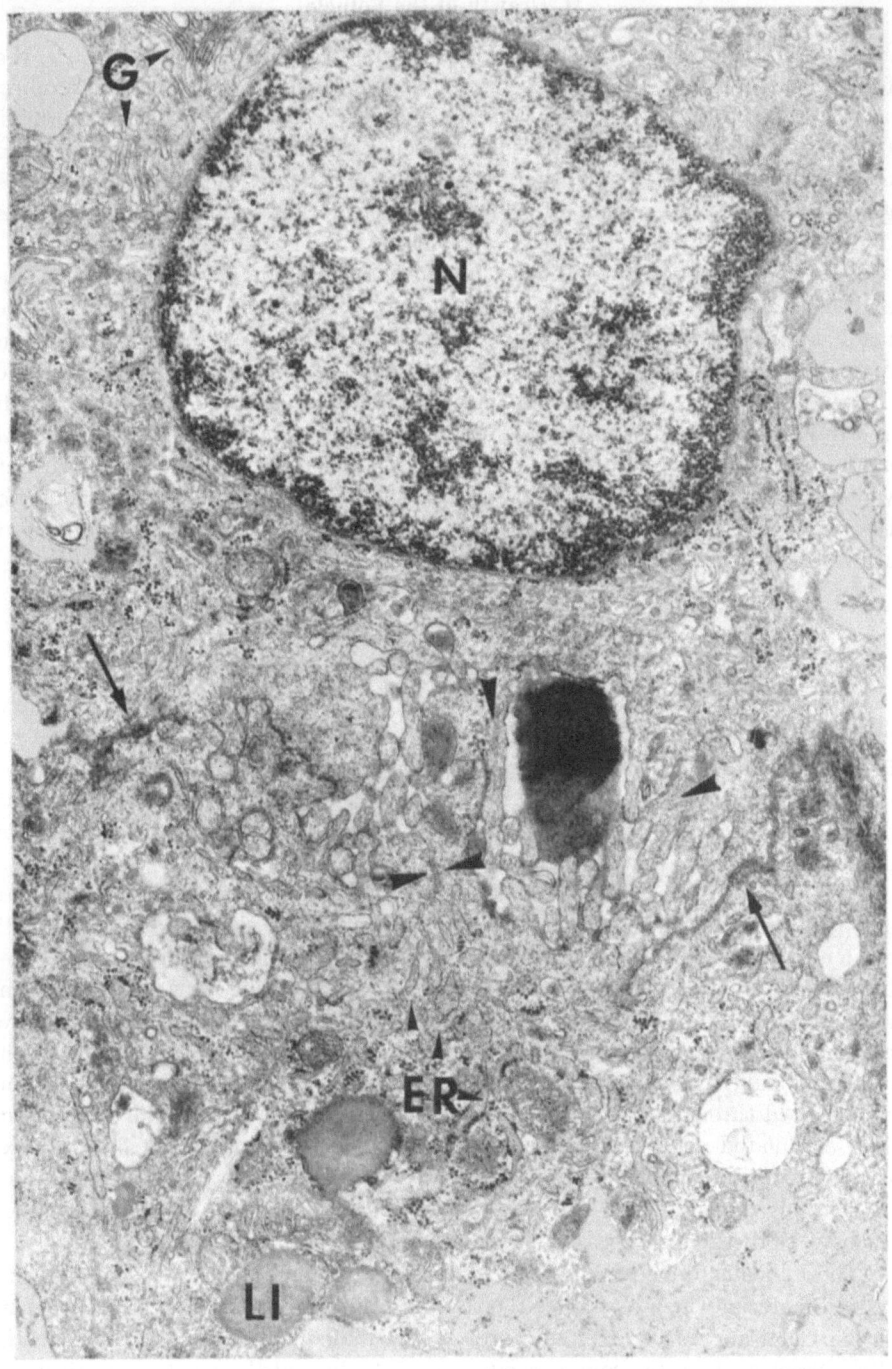

Fig. 9. TSH-stimulated culture, 36 h. Dilution of the dense follicular material; core of microfilaments in the microvilli (▶); E. R. cisternae (*ER*), reaching directly into the follicular
lumen (▶◀); lipid inclusion (*LI*); adult junctional complexes (→); nucleus (*N*); Golgi
apparatus (*G*). ×30,000

D. Growth of the Follicle

The growth of the follicle takes place progressively. After 3 days culture, the follicle becomes about spherical and is composed of 4–6 epithelial cells, surrounding a lumen about 10 μ in diameter. We never observed any mitosis in the cultures. Of course, dissociated and in vitro cultured cells can divide when put into a medium containing 30–40% Calf serum for 12 h (Fayet, unpublished), but the aggregates growth and the enlargement of follicular lumen do not seem to result from the division of the constituting cells.

At the beginning, the follicular lumen is almost completely filled with an extremely osmiophilic material, which at very high magnifications seems to be made up of oriented granules, filaments or tubules measuring about 60 Å in diameter (Fig. 7b). After several h in culture this material seems to become diluted and forms very fine anastomosed trabeculae anchored on the microvilli and interlinking them (Figs. 9, 10); it could represent a glycocalyx-type material at the apical surface of the cell. The elaboration of this material, the density of which is much higher than that of thyroid colloid, seems to be closely related to the phenomena of microvilli morphogenesis, which can be very easily observed after 6 to 12 h of culture.

E. The Cells Reassociated after Several Days of Culture

After several days, tangential sections of stimulated cultures (Fig. 11a) show numerous large cell clumps in which follicles at all stages of maturation can be found. Spreading of the cells and accentuation of their polarity results progressively in their polygonal shape in sections. Some cells can measure 20 μ long and 6–7 μ wide. However, several smaller, less frequent, completely isolated cells conserving a rounded or oval shape can also be found.

The nucleus of the reassociated cells is larger (7 μ in diameter) and has several small indentations. The chromatin is again very finely dispersed with a small condensation along the nuclear membrane. This appearance is the same as that in the in vivo gland. The nucleolus is often very visible and very large, and can measure up to 2 μ in diameter. In the TSH-stimulated cells and especially in the presence of hydrocortisone, nuclear constituents seem to separate from each other and clumps of dense interchromatin granules are found in contact with them or dispersed throughout the nuclear sap. In the reassociated or non-reassociated TSH-stimulated cells nuclear bodies (1–3 per nucleus) measuring 3,000 Å are very frequently found. Their structure, which can be either very finely granular or filamentous depending on the plane of section, and a clear surrounding allows them to be distinguished easily enough from the nucleoplasm (Fig. 11a, b).

The follicular lumen is lined by microvilli and contains a very slightly contrasted material which resembles the thyroid colloid; the very active components of the Golgi apparatus are found around the follicular lumen. Numerous small clear vesicles separate from the edges of 7–8 distended saccules constituting Golgi dictyosomes. The Golgi area is surrounded by several either small-sized and oval or large and rounded shaped dense bodies. It contains small bundles of microfilaments, numerous microtubules and one or two centrioles with voluminous satellite bodies and one or two sometimes very long ciliary rootlets, recognizable by their periodical 350 Å spacing cross-striation (Figs. 7a, 8, 11a).

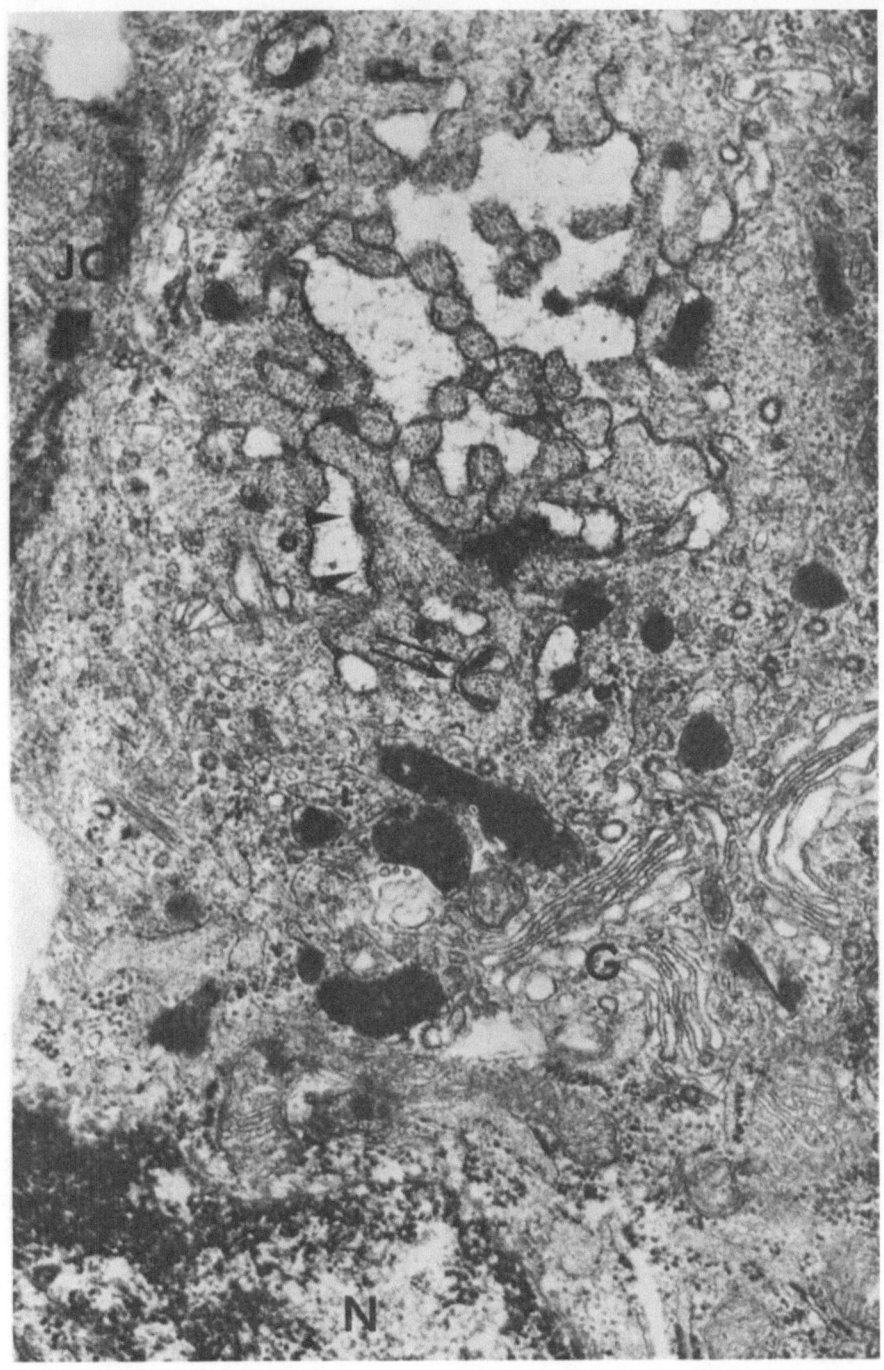

Fig. 10. TSH-stimulated culture, 36 h. Dispersion of follicular material into very fine filaments; at the tip of the microvilli (▶) the membrane becomes denser; horse-shoe shaped vesicles (⇉); vesicles containing a material of high electron density (→), budding at the Golgi apparatus (*G*); junctional complex (*JC*); nucleus (*N*). ×30,000

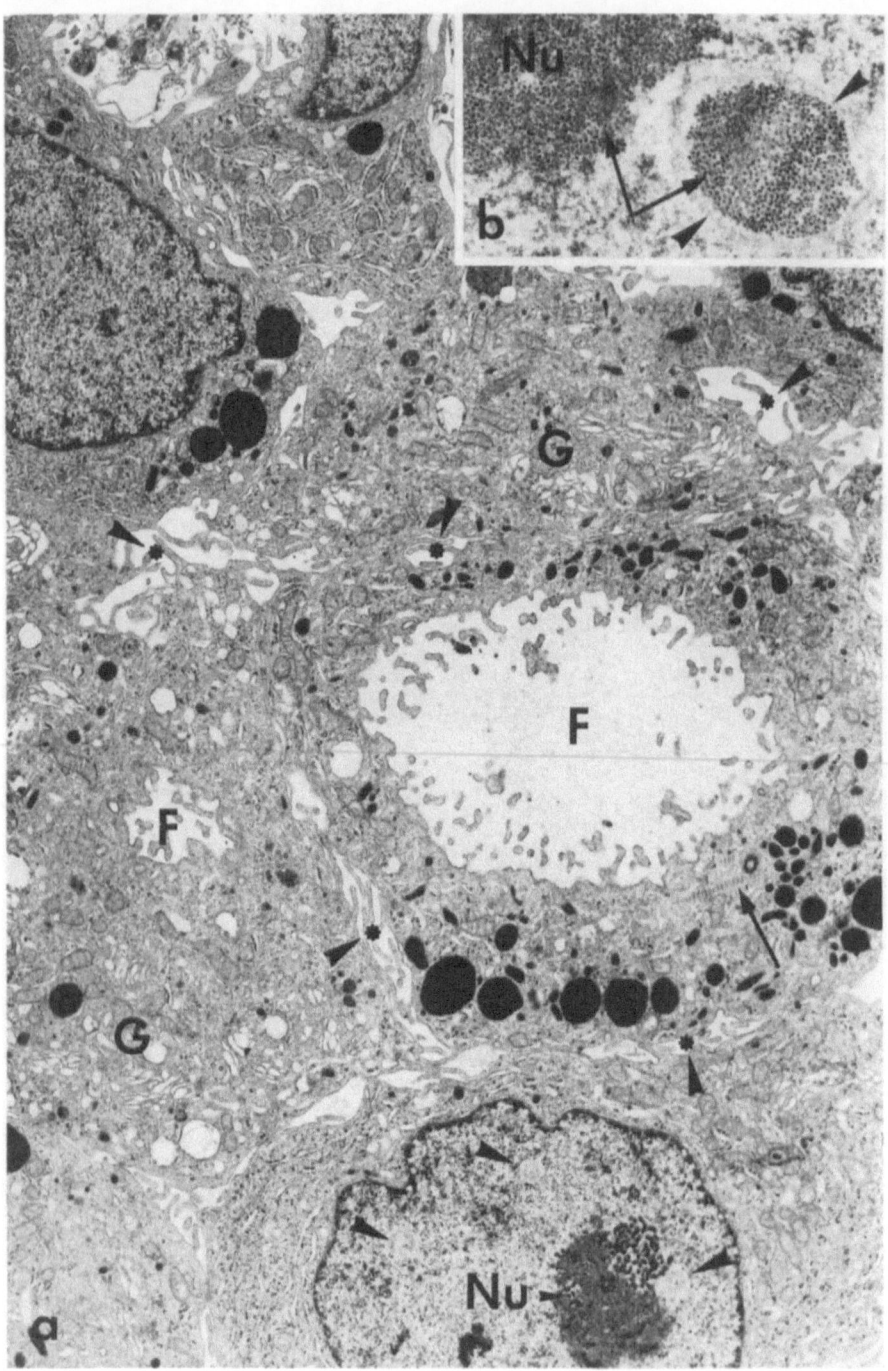

Fig. 11a a. b. TSH-stimulated culture in the presence of hydrocortisone, 6 days. (a) General view; "intracytoplasmic" follicular lumina (F); intercellular spaces (▶✳); numerous nuclear bodies (▶) next to the nucleolus (Nu); centriole and ciliary rootlet ($\rightarrow$). ×8,800. (b) Nucleolus (Nu) and granular nuclear body surrounded by a fibrillar capsule (▶); compare the size of the nucleolar granules with those composing the nuclear body ($\rightarrow$). ×30,000

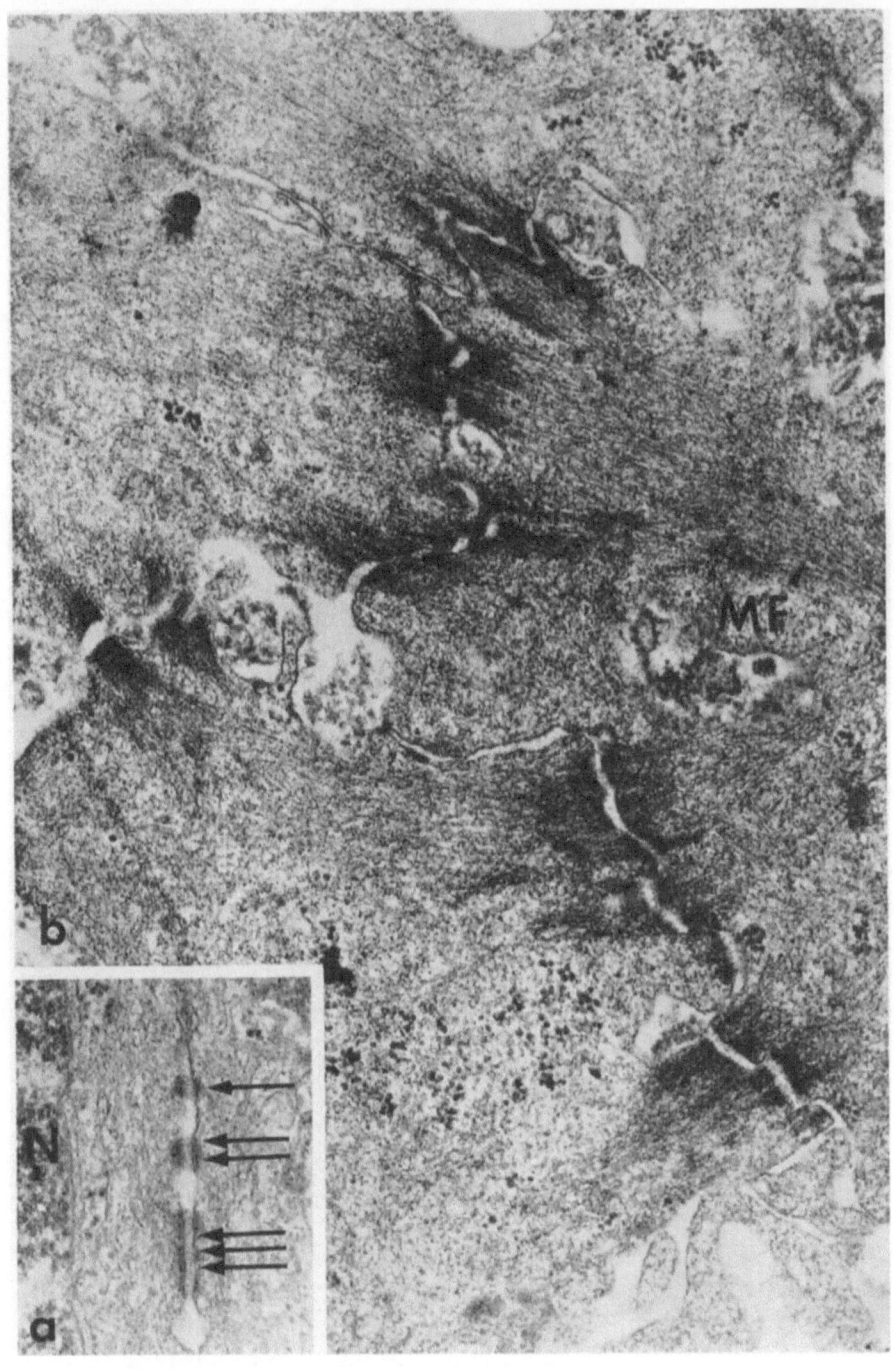

Fig. 12a a. b. Control culture, 60 h. (a) Successive stages in the formation of the desmosomes; non-reassociated cells. (b) Adult desmosomes linked by microfilaments (*MF*) (compare with a); reassociated cells. ×50,000

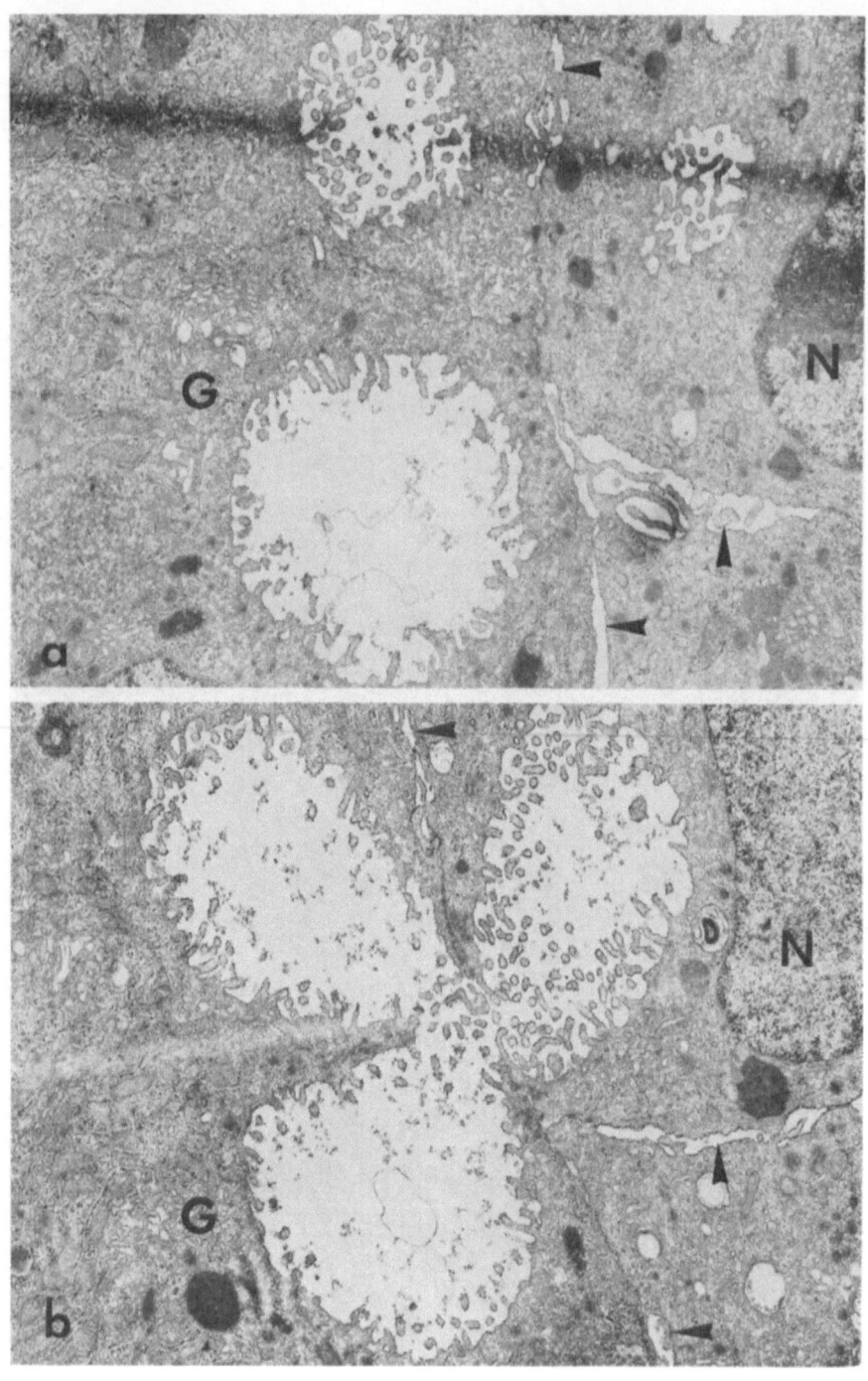

Fig. 13 a a. b. TSH-stimulated culture, 4 days. Serial sections: (a) image of "intracytoplasmic" follicles; intercellular spaces (▶); nucleus (N); Golgi apparatus (G). (b) Clover-leaf image. ×12,000

This frequency of ciliary structures appears as a general feature of cultured thyroid cells even when not reassociated. All stages in the formation of cilia can thus be observed. It begins with the presence in the center of the Golgi region of a vacuole at first very flattened, which afterwards incurvates, becoming more or less hemispherical, and then comes into contact by its concave face with microtubules inserted in a basal body; then this ciliary vesicle progressively approaches the apical pole. It finally results in an often very long cilium bathing in the thyroid colloid. Sections perpendicular to the axis of the cilium show that its structure is often imperfect; both axial tubules and sometimes even several peripheral doublets can be missing.

The endoplasmic reticulum appears in the form of a network of anastomosed channels very frequently surrounding the mitochondria. The cisternae, which are seldom distended, contain a material of low contrast. Numerous free ribosomes are still dispersed in the hyaloplasm.

The plasmalemma, except on the free surface which bounds the follicular cavity, has numerous digitiform extensions occupying the entire intercellular space and intermingled with those of adjacent cells. These extensions attain a great length on the side of the culture in contact with the plastic support of the Falcon dish.

Short desmosomes (500 Å long) laterally unite the cells. At the apical pole an adult junctional complex isolates the follicular lumen from the lateral intercellular spaces. This complex measures 1.5 μ and comprises a zonula occludens, a zonula adherens and one or several desmosomes.

Next to these adult follicles all the previously described stages of follicular maturation may be found in small aggregates comprising 2 or 3 cells which up to then have not reassociated.

IV. Other Elements in the Culture

A. The C Cells

We have never encountered C cells mingled with reassociated or non-reassociated follicular cells. It should be kept in mind that C cells are very scarce in the Pig's thyroid (Young, 1966).

B. Connective Tissue Components

The free connective tissue cells, namely mastocytes, lymphocytes and macrophages, can only be recognized during the early hours of culture. These cells seem to be masked by epithelial proliferation and follicular reassociation. It must be noted, however, that at the end of the first week, the macrophages reappear when the reconstituted follicles break up and phagocytose the degenerated epithelial cells (Mauchamp, unpublished observation).

On the other hand, collagen fibrils which are rather short and isolated from each other are frequently observed between the thyroid cells. Similarly to what occurs for cells, this collagen generally disappears within 24 h. Nevertheless, in the first culture examined, numerous fibers were still present after 36 h culture in the absence of TSH; this abundance of collagen corresponded to a very conspicuous follicular reassociation and a very differentiated aspect of the thyroid cells. These

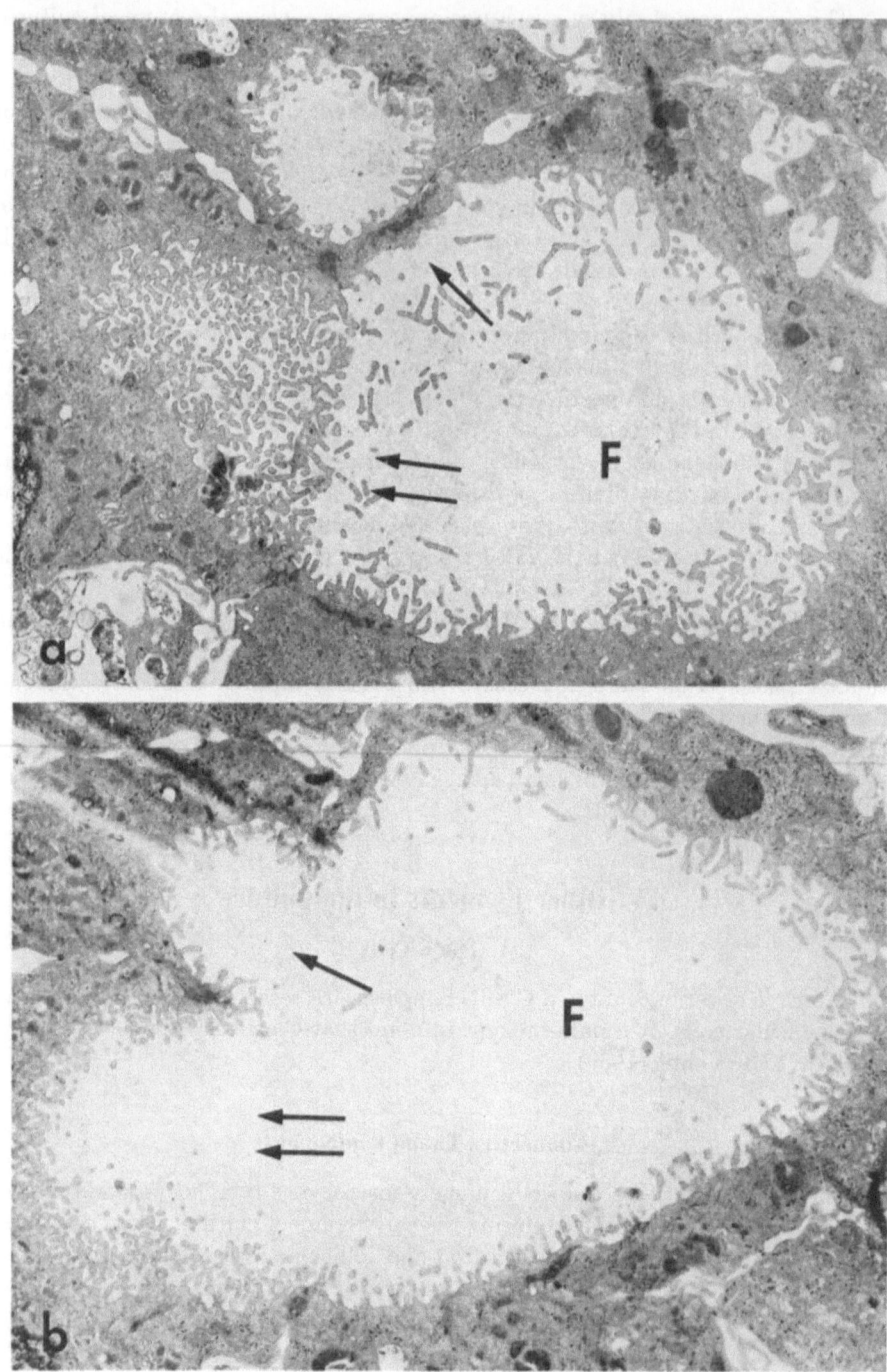

Fig. 14a a. b. TSH-stimulated culture in the presence of hydrocortisone, 60 h. Serial sections:
(a) "intracytoplasmic microfollicle" (→) next to a second cavity (⇉) which opens into a
large-sized follicle (F). (b) The two small-sized follicular cavities opening into the large one (F).
×8,800

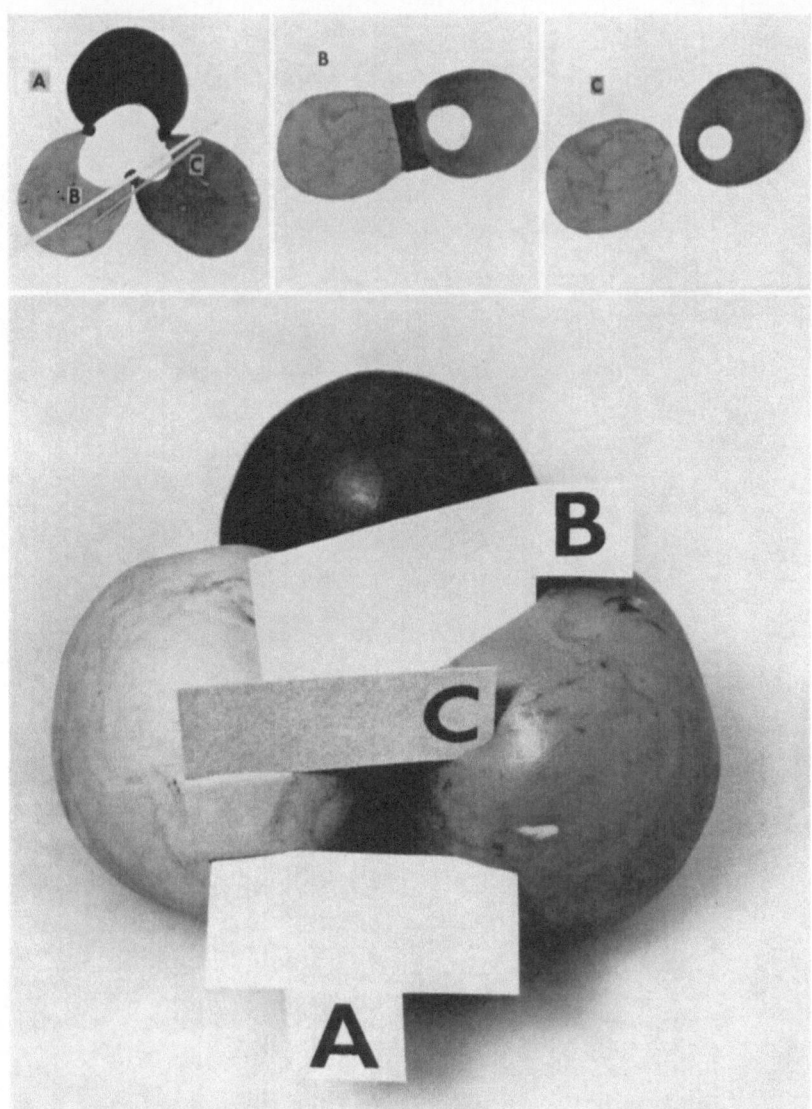

Fig. 15. Follicular models sectioned in three planes, A. B, C: Plane of section A: horizontal: follicle appears clover-leaf shaped. Plane of section B: vertical perpendicular to plane A: "intracytoplasmic follicle" next to the cell junction. Plane of section C: vertical perpendicular to plane A: isolated "intracytoplasmic follicle"

connective fibers, however, do not show any organization around the isolated or reassociated cells. Moreover, we did not find any fibrocytes in the three fragments of this culture examined with the electron microscope.

C. Basal Lamina

In all the cultures studied, no basal lamina can be observed around isolated cells or at the basal pole of reassociated cells.

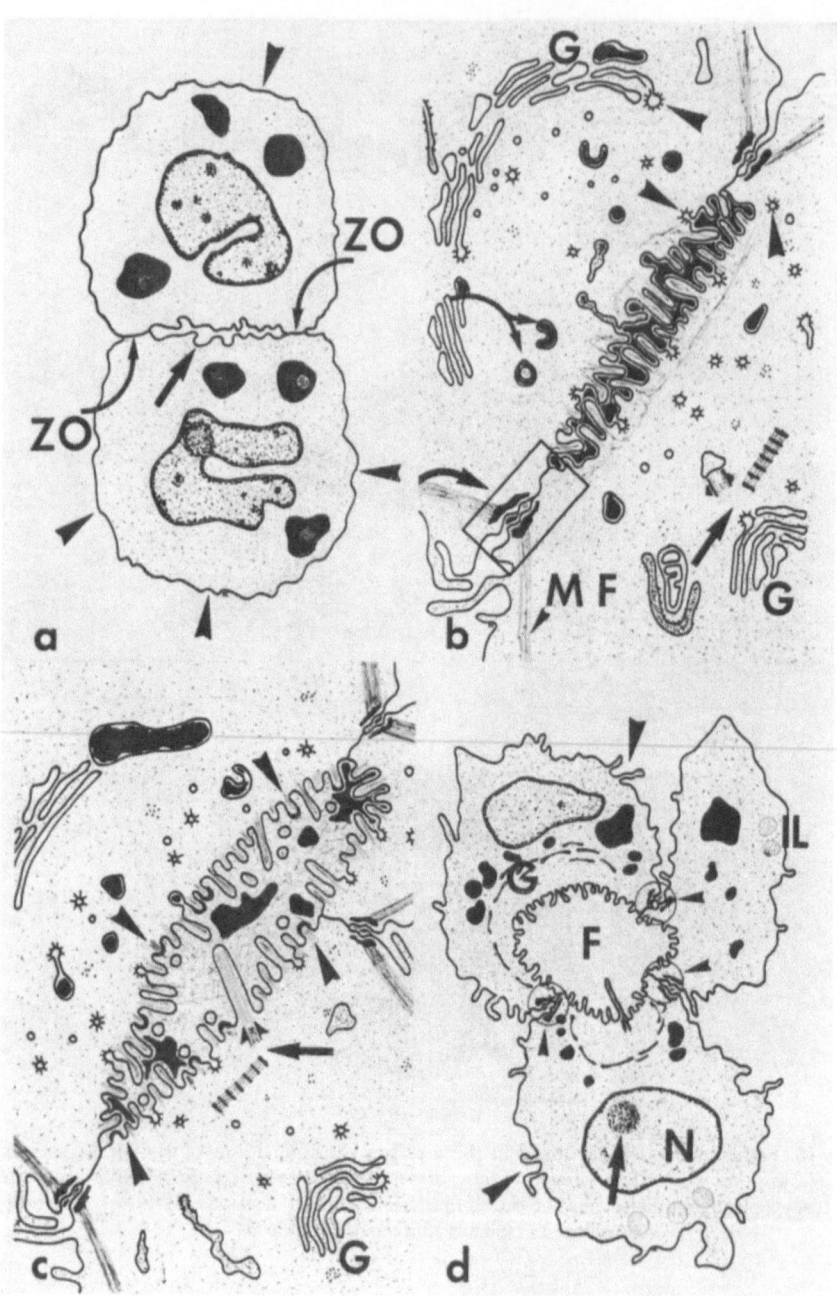

Fig. 16a—d. Stages in the formation of follicles *in vitro* by dissociated thyroid cells in culture. (a) Reconstruction of the zonula occludens (*ZO*) between two cells, absence of lateral and basal cell extensions (▶); indented nuclei. (b) Appearance of microvilli and dense follicular material; maturation of the cell junctions; appearance of cilia (→); double population of "coated" Golgi and endocytotic vesicles (▶); appearance of horse-shoe shaped vesicles possibly arising from the Golgi apparatus (*G*); microfilaments (*MF*). (c) Dispersion of the dense intrafollicular material; adjunction of a third cell to the follicular cavity; appearance of the cell coat and the apex of microvilli containing a core of microfilaments (▶). (d) Growth of the follicular lumen giving rise to a clover-leaf shape between three adult cell junctions (▶○);

In conclusion, thyroid cells isolated by trypsinization from adult Pig glands and cultured in vitro very rapidly reconstitute typical follicular structures. After 15 min stimulation by TSH, the cells again group together, make contact and partition by means of a zonula occludens (Fig. 16a) a closed space into which characteristic microvilli develop and wherein an osmiophilic material accumulates (Fig. 16b). The follicular lumen then progressively grows larger and probably additional cells join those already reassociated (Fig. 16c, d). The same process also takes place within the same lapse of time in cultures not stimulated by TSH. However in the latter case after about 4 days the cultures lose the acquired follicular structure and form a true monolayer.

New cells reassociate during the growth of the follicles constituted in the first h, and this process still goes on for some time, so that even after more than a week of culture in the presence of TSH narrow lumina of newly formed follicles at various stages of maturation can be observed next to large follicles bearing numerous epithelial cells.

Discussion

I. Biochemical Aspects of Follicular Reassociation in Cultured Thyroid Cells

A. Reaggregation of Dissociated Cells: General Review of Known Biological Systems

Since the early work of Wilson (1907–1911), a great many authors have studied the fate in vitro or after grafts in vivo of all sorts of cells dissociated by mechanical means, by substraction of calcium and/or magnesium ions, by enzymatic action or by a combination of these techniques (cf. reviews by Harris, 1964; Sigot, 1965; Moscona and Wilmer, 1966).

1. The Example of Dictyostelium Discoideum

The research on Dictyostelium discoideum constitute a summary of all the problems posed by the phenomena of cell reaggregation. When this Amoeba is placed in a medium rich in nutritive elements, it proliferates in the form of a culture of cells isolated from each other which divide by mitosis. When the environmental conditions become unfavorable for growth, Dictyostelium cells reaggregate forming a pseudo-plasmodial mass wherein spores differentiate.

(1) What is the mechanism which allows the cells to reaggregate?

(2) What are the various means ensuring adhesion between the cells in the pseudoplasmodium?

2. Reaggregation Mechanisms

a) In Dictyostelium Discoideum

The reaggregation of cells isolated from Dictyostelium discoideum is induced by a chemotaxic factor, acrasine (general review: Cohen and Robertson, 1971).

---

appearance of lateral and basal cytoplasmic extensions; nuclear turgescence and a large nucleolus (→); lipid inclusions at the basal pole (IL)

Acrasine is in fact 3'–5' cyclic AMP produced by the cells (Barkley, 1969) and released at regular intervals into the medium by the amoebae at the time of aggregation (Gerisch, 1968). This phenomenon has been reproduced experimentally (Robertson et al., 1972).

b) In Other Species

Similarly, specific aggregation factors synthesized and released into the culture medium by previously dissociated cells have been described during re-aggregation of sponge cells and cells derived from Invertebrate and Vertebrate embryos. They are glycoprotein molecules and their form has been observed in some cases with the electron microscope (for the Sponge: Moscona, 1963; Humphreys, 1965; Muller and Zahn, 1973; Henkart et al., 1973; Cauldwell et al., 1973; for the Urchin: Tonegawa, 1973; for the neuroretina of Chick embryo: Lilien and Moscona, 1967; Richmond et al., 1968; Daday, 1972; for embryonic Chick and Mouse brain cells: Garber, 1972; Balsamo and Lilien, 1974).

In some cell types other macromolecules containing nucleotide derivatives were described. This group of aggregation promoting factors, however, might originate from the chromosomes of the cells destroyed during isolation (Steinberg, 1963; Iwig et al., 1973).

c) The Specificity of Aggregation Promoting Factors

3'–5' cyclic AMP is the chemical mediator for reaggregation of Dictyostelium discoideum cells and the cells of 3 other species of Amoebae, but it is not common to all known species of Amoeba (Bonner et al., 1972). The same species and cell type specificity exists for the glycoprotein aggregation factors in higher organisms and corresponds to the relative species specificity observed in Amoebae.

In answer to the first question it seems that dissociated cells produce a specific material which brings about their aggregation in vitro by a process similar to the chemotaxis demonstrated in Dictyostelium discoideum.

3. Mechanisms of Cell Adhesion

a) In Dictyostelium Discoideum

The mechanism or mechanisms allowing the cells of the Amoeba to adhere together and keep the pseudoplasmodial architecture is almost totally unknown. The presence of calcium ions is indispensable (Mason et al., 1971) as is the case in many systems. At the beginning of aggregation new antigenic sites appear in the cell surface. These sites might play a role in intercellular adhesion (Beug et al., 1973).

b) In Other Species

In the other cell systems studied several theories have been proposed to account for the adhesion of cells to each other.

Early authors (Tyler, 1947; Weiss, 1958) postulated that cell surfaces could be joined to each other by macromolecular complexes. The interactions between these molecules might be comparable either to those between antigen and antibody during the formation of the immune complex (recently interactions between membrane antigens and the specific factor of aggregation have been described: Pessac and Defendi, 1972; Balsamo and Lilien, 1974), or to those between an enzyme and its substrate (the role of glycosyl-transferases has beeen proposed: Roseman, 1970; Roth, 1973). According to this hypothesis these macromolecular complexes might contain proteins analogous to actomyosin which would cause the adhesion of fibroblasts in vitro (Jones and Kemp, 1970), as well as of skeletal muscle cells and hepatocytes after trypsinization (Garnett et al., 1973). Biochemical and immunohistochemical studies (Booyse and Rafelson, 1972) seem to have established that this is the role played by thrombostenin in the adhesion of platelets. Likewise these macromolecular interactions might explain the specificity of cellular adhesion (Roth, 1968).

Contrary to this, Curtiss (1962) suggested that cell adhesion is due to purely physical phenomena involving electrostatic (London van der Waals' forces) and repulsive forces due e. g. to ions adsorbed on the cell membranes surface.

In answer to the second question it therefore seems that at least two types of mechanisms can account for the adhesion of cells to each other in aggregates in vivo or in vitro: a) physical mechanisms involving electrostatic properties of cell membranes, b) active biological mechanisms requiring reciprocal interactions between macromolecules situated at the cell surface.

B. Reaggregation and Reassociation of Isolated Thyroid Cells

1. Analogy with Known Systems

As in other biological systems studied, it seems that the reaggregation process can be distinguished from adhesion and reassociation of previously dissociated adult thyroid cells.

a) Reaggregation Promoting Factor

A glycoprotein factor promoting aggregation of thyroid cells in 6 h is at present being studied (Giraud, 1975).

b) Cellular Adhesion and Metabolic Activity

Though there are numerous modifications in the cell surface due to the action of trypsin (review by Steinberg et al., 1973), repair of the plasma membrane, which is indispensable for the establishment of cell relationships and recovery of metabolic activity and normal function, takes place very rapidly after trypsinization. Within 15 or 20 min after trypsinization aggregates comprising 2 or 3 cells are formed (Mallette and Anthony, 1966). Furthermore, 2 h after their isolation and start of their culture, thyroid cells are able to phagocytize latex particles (Rodesch et al., 1970).

Therefore it is nor surprising that the first images of reassociation are seen as soon as after 15 min in culture.

2. Role of TSH in Reaggregation and Follicular Reassociation in Vitro

a) Data from the Literature

The results obtained by various authors appear contradictory. According to some, follicular reassociation is observed, as well with the light microscope (Kerkoff et al., 1964; Fayet and Tixier, 1967; Kalderon and Wittner, 1967; Fayet et al., 1970) as with the electron microscope (Fayet et al., 1971), only in the presence of TSH.

Others, investigating the fate of isolated thyroid cells *in vitro* without stimulation by TSH, did not observe any follicular structure even after several h of culture (Shimazaki et al., 1967; Tixier-Vidal et al., 1969).

Others, in the same experimental conditions, noted the appearance of typical but small-sized follicles (Mallette and Anthony, 1966; Neve et al,. 1968; Spooner, 1970).

b) Reasons for these Contradictions

The contradictions result from differences in the conditions of observations:

first, the time elapsed before examination of the stimulated or non-stimulated culture. In fact, adult (or embryonic) thyroid cells, dissociated and cultured in the absence of TSH, do reassociate but only during the first 3 or 4 days of culture, after which time the follicles disappear and the culture becomes a monolayer;

second, the order of magnitude of observed details, in other words the use of light or electron microscopy, is most important. The size of the microfollicles present in the control or stimulated cultures after several h is at the limit of resolution of the light microscope especially if they contain only few colloid and if this has abnormal staining affinities. These microfollicles are then visible only after a careful examination with the electron microscope.

Moreover, thyroid cells in culture present considerable deformations; some are annular and contain a cavity which is devoid of microvilli and sometimes filled by cellular debris. This cavity seems to result from the formation of giant lysosomes which have either been excreted by the cells or removed during the processing for electron microscopy. These cavities, which are sometimes large-sized, can be mistaken for follicular lumina especially when examined in phase contrast. This is why the follicles present in the non-stimulated cultures cannot be seen by the light microscope during the first days.

c) Conclusion

Since follicular reassociation occurs in control cultures less than 4 days old and in stimulated cultures, it seems therefore that exogenic thyrotropin added to the culture medium is not the factor inducing the morphogenetic phenomena. This is confirmed by the fact that freshly trypsinized thyroid cells bear very few membrane receptor sites for thyrotropin and therefore cannot respond to this specific stimulation. Moreover, reconstitution of TSH specific cell receptors occurs only after 24 h culture (Lissitzky et al., 1973). Nevertheless TSH seems indispensable for the maintenance and growth of the follicular structure, after 3 or 4 days' culture.

Morphogenesis of thyroid follicles in vitro can be compared with development of thyroid gland in vivo. Thus, though the anterior pituitary very early contains TSH (Almquist et al., 1970) and though injection of TSH into embryonic Chick thyroids is followed by the appearing of follicles (Boyd, 1964), it seems that follicular morphogenesis in the thyroid gland occurs independently from TSH. This is supported by hypophysectomy and encephalectomy experiments (Jost, 1953) as well as by observation of associated cultures of fragments of fetal thyroid and pituitary gland (Tixier-Vidal, 1958). However, follicular structure maintenance and growth of follicles, in vivo (Bearn, 1966) or in vitro (Tixier-Vidal, 1958), require the presence of TSH.

3. Other Factors that Could Be Responsible for Follicular Morphogenesis in Vitro

a) Endogenous TSH

Endogenous (Pig) TSH fixed to the cell membranes at the time of isolation could, if not destroyed during trypsinization, induce reaggregation and follicular reassociation since thyroid cells inactivate TSH more slowly in vitro than in vivo (Boeynaems et al., 1973). Nevertheless, this seems rather unlikely since 65% of TSH membrane receptors are destroyed by 1 min trypsin (Lissitzky et al., 1973). It is also possible that the complex formed between the membrane receptor and the TSH molecule can resist enzymatic hydrolysis and that the hormone keeps some biological activity when the free receptor is destroyed by trypsin.

b) 3′–5′ Cyclic AMP (cAMP)

3′–5′ cAMP is the second hormonal messenger of thyrotropin hormone and it mimics the metabolic effects of TSH in vitro (Fayet and Lissitzky, 1970; Lissitzky et al., 1971). It is rather unlikely that cAMP could be responsible for reaggregation and follicular reassociation since it would have to be released and remain in the culture medium without being hydrolysed. Moreover, cAMP inhibits adhesion in vitro of tumor cells of Ehrlich's ascites on protein-coated plastic surfaces (Weiss, 1973) and aggregation of trypsin-dissociated embryonic Quail hepatocytes cultured in vitro (Kuroda, 1974).

c) Other Thyroid Molecules

Other molecules liberated into the culture medium by destroyed cells could play a role, for instance thyroid DNA, by analogy with other embryonic tissues (Steinberg, 1963), or total thyroid RNA which in vitro has an action comparable to TSH (Chernly and Mu, 1973). In fact, the synthesis of RNA and particularly m-RNA is indispensable for reassociation as is shown by the action of metabolic inhibitors (Lissitzky et al., 1971). Thyroglobulin, liberated by cellular death or synthesized and secreted into the culture medium, might also play a role for it has a TSH-like activity on some aspects of thyroid metabolism (Burke and Szabo, 1972). But these authors used a much higher quantity of thyroglobulin than the levels detected in the culture medium of thyroid cells. Furthermore, thyroglobulin does not seem to have any effect, at the light microscope level, on follicular reassociation in culture (Giraud, 1975).

d) Connective Tissue Elements

Connective elements, though rarely observed, are present right at the beginning of the culture, and they might influence somewhat the development of cultures (Kerkoff et al., 1964; Fayet et al., 1970). In many embryonic organs specific interactions between the mesenchyme and the neighbouring epithelium have been described. A specific action of thyroid connective tissue on differentiation and follicular morphogenesis of embryonic thyroid gland has been shown (Hilfer et al., 1967; Hilfer, 1968). We ourselves observed in one case exuberant growth of a culture in which numerous collagen fibres happened to be present; this may be merely coincidental and, though obviously suggestive, cannot be interpreted as significant for a specific interaction.

In addition to these factors rather specific of thyroid tissue, non-specific molecules contained in the Calf serum supplementing the culture medium, even if only protein or mucopolysaccharides (Pessac et al., 1973), could attenuate the effects of trypsin (Steinberg et al., 1973). Our cultures did not provide any proof of this presumed role of one or other of these factors.

4. Conclusion

The fate of adult thyroid cells in vitro seems to be comparable in all respects to that of embryonic cells as studied in vivo and in vitro:

the reaggregate under the influence of a glycoproteic factor analogous to those described in other biological systems;

the mechanisms of adhesion and factors promoting cell differentiation in the follicles are still totally unknown;

the maintenance and growth of the follicles require the presence of TSH during embryonic life and in culture, whereas thyrotropin does not seem to be indispensable to the building of follicular architecture as is evidenced by the early stages of the gland histogenesis, by the differentiation under the influence of a specific mesenchymatous factor of grafted embryonic thyroid cells and by the presence of numerous follicles in early, non stimulated cultures.

Besides, it is probable that the interactions between cells in culture and the substrate surface on which they grow play a very large, though poorly known role in follicular reassociation. For instance, it has been shown (Mauchamp and Fayet, 1974) that freshly isolated cells may rearrange into follicles when grown on a sheath of either collagen or glutaraldehyde-treated gelatin on which they do not adhere, and that cells from a culture which has reached the monolayer state after 1 week in TSH containing medium recover ability to constitute follicles when placed on such a non-adhesive substrate.

The process of follicular morphogenesis is likely to involve several types of different mechanisms, the most part of which are but little understood.

II. Ultrastructural Aspects of Follicular Reassociation

A. Cells after Trypsinization

Morphological studies confirm that trypsin has two distinct targets in the cells.

1. Plasmalemma Modifications

The main changes noticed after isolation of the cells are in the plasmalemma (Figs. 2, 4). The cells become round or oval-shaped and lose most of their cytoplasmic protrusions. The same has been reported in other cell types (Dalen and Todd, 1971).

Cell isolation is never quite complete, so that numerous junctional complexes resist enzymatic hydrolysis and intact follicular fragments are found in the culture. The same observations have been made by other authors (Hilfer and Hilfer, 1966; Neve et al., 1969). Such unequal sensitivity to trypsin could correspond to a biochemical difference between two almost identical cell junctions, as is the case for desmosomes (Borysenko and Revel, 1973).

2. Cytoplasmic Modifications

Furthermore, the transformation of some cytoplasmic organelles can result from the direct action of trypsin. It has been shown by immunofluorescence and radioautography of labeled trypsin that the enzyme penetrates the cytoplasm (and even the nucleus), probably by a process of endocytosis, and keeps its lytic activity (Hodges et al., 1973). Consequently, trypsin itself might be responsible for an increase of lysosomal dense bodies, vacuolisation of the E. R. and modifications observed in the bound versus free ribosomes ratio (Hosick and Strohman, 1971).

B. Follicular Reassociation

1. Reconstitution of the Cell Junctions

The cell junction reconstitution, as observed with the electron microscope, is the first morphological evidence of cell adhesion taking place at the molecular level, and it is the first stage of follicular reassociation. Evolution of the means of this cell adhesion is comparable to that observed in embryonic or in vitro cultured epithelial cells (see below).

a) Cell Contacts

In small aggregates formed very early in the cultures differentiated cell junctions are absent. The most straightlined segments, which might constitute the beginning of a means of union (Curtiss, 1962, Fig. 4), can be noted in discrete zones of the plasma membrane in adjacent cells.

b) Zonula Occludens

An annular zonula occludens joins the two or three newly reassociated cells and isolates the early follicular cleft. As has been previously reported during the development of the choroid epithelium (Doolin and Birge, 1969) and of the telencephalic capillaries endothelium (Delforme, 1972), the zonula occludens is formed by the plasma membranes progressively coming together at several neighbouring points (Fig. 5a, b), then by the fusion in these discrete zones of the membrane. The adult-type zonula occludens results from new zones of fusion appearing between the first ones and from their subsequent extension until complete continuity is established (Fig. 6a, b).

c) Adult Junctional Complex

The appearance of other elements of the junctional complex, such as zonula adherens and desmosomes, takes place several hours later in the cultures.

Many authors have studied desmosome differentiation during the development of epithelial cells of fowl blastoderm in vivo or after dissociation by trypsin (Overton, 1962) of corneal epidermis in culture (Blumcke et al., 1968), of avian choroidal epithelium (Doolin and Birge, 1969), and during cicatrization of the epidermis in vivo (Krawczyk and Wilgram, 1973). The appearance of the desmosome takes place through three successive stages:

(1) the condensation of an electron-dense material situated between two juxtaposed membrane segments; (2) the adjacent cytoplasm becomes dense; (3) the development of a large network of microfilaments anchored to this dense cytoplasmic area.

The same mechanism seems to be involved in cultures of thyroid cells. As has been observed during cicatrization of the epidermis, the intercellular material often presents a filamentous structure oriented perpendicularly to the membranes. The interval of time between trypsinization and appearance of the desmosomes (about 12 h) is comparable to that observed in Fowl blastoderm. They are present both in control and stimulated cultures, but they only reach a large size in the presence of TSH or in reassociated cells (Fig. 12a, b). The stages of zonula adherens formation are the same as for the desmosome except for lacking of the last stage, i. e. the development of a network of microfilaments anchored to the dense plaque.

The sequence of formation of these means of union in adult thyroid cell cultures favors the theory that these three cell junctions also represent a sequence of attachment mechanisms between the cells (Kelly and Luft, 1966).

Thus in the adult follicles the junctional complex associates the three elements described. We did not observe the absence of zonula adherens, known as sometimes lacking in Rat thyroid cells (Farquhar and Palade, 1963).

The union between cells seems to be necessary for the recovery of functional activity by the cell organelles; in addition some transfer of information is likely to take place between the cells via certain junctions (Loewenstein, 1967, 1973; Azarnia et al., 1974).

d) The Problem of Reconstitution of Cell Polarity

The question arises whether thyroid cells, during their reassociation, use the same portions of their plasmalemma by which they were joined in vivo; in other words whether they keep beyond their ultrastructural appearance a polarity at the level of the membrane macromolecules necessary for the formation of cell junctions.

It seems that the cells can reassociate at random at any point of their plasmalemma and that they reconstitute new means of union instead of using the remnants of those which have been more or less destroyed during trypsinization. This is obviously the case in fragments of the follicular epithelium present in the cultures during the first hours: images of reassociation with formation of a zonula occludens are observed between 2 cells, one of which remains linked at another part of its membrane to a third cell by an adult and certainly pre-existing junctional complex. The lumen of the new follicle is thus derived from what was previously the lateral cell space (Fig. 5a).

Likewise when corneal epithelial cells reaggregate their membrane still bears after isolation several residual hemi-desmosomes, but the sites of the new cell junctions are different and perfect juxtaposition of two hemi-desmosomes situated in two adjacent cells is only rarely observed during the first days of culture (Overton, 1973).

2. Cytoplasmic and Nuclear Modifications

The ultrastructural modifications in the Golgi apparatus and the R. E. R. are related to a high activity of synthesis particularly of thyroglobulin, as is shown by biochemical studies. Nonetheless, it seems that thyroid cells cultured in the presence of TSH do not completely recover their former morphologic appearance. This is most noticeable for the ribosomes, many of which remain isolated in the hyaloplasma (Figs. 6b, 7a, 8–10).

There seems to be a much higher degree of autolytic activity than that observed in vivo. This could be due on the one hand to the action of trypsin and, on the other hand to the presence in the cytoplasm of non utilized organelles, especially free ribosomes. It might also be related to the increased level of intracellular cAMP in the case of TSH-stimulated cells, since cAMP can bring about an increase in autophagy in many types of cells e. g. in hepatic cells (Shelburne et al., 1973). The target-like images already mentioned and perhaps indicative of such a process have been observed in cultures of dissociated embryonic thyroid cells (Spooner, 1970).

Numerous nuclear bodies are very frequently present in the TSH-stimulated cells. These nuclear inclusions are related to an increase in protein synthesis (Simar, 1969) and arise from the nucleolus (Dupuy-Coin and Bouteille, 1972) with which they have a close relationship (Fig. 11 a, b).

3. Morphogenesis of the Microvilli

Cultures of thyroid cells allow the study of the morphogenesis of the microvilli which ruffle the apical pole of adult cells.

Three mechanisms have been proposed to account for the formation of the microvilli:

(1) The microvilli arise by pinking out of the apical pole by elongated vesicles which merge into each other perpendicularly to the plasmalemma. The faces of these fused vesicles constitute the lateral faces of the microvilli. This seems to be the case for retinal cells in Planarians and for Rat kidney cells (Röhlich, 1962).

(2) The microvilli arise from budding of the cell surface related to expanding bundles of microfilaments which become their axial core. This is the case in intestinal cells of Insects (Van Lennep, 1964), of metamorphosing Amphibia (Hourdry, 1969), of the Rat (Shaw-Dunn, 1967), and in BHK cells in culture (Follet and Goldman, 1970).

(3) The membrane of the microvilli arises from the fusion with the apical plasmalemma of a vesicle originating from the Golgi apparatus and containing an electron-dense material. The form of this vesicle is variable, either rounded, twisted or sometimes horse-shoe shaped. These vesicles have been described in intestinal epithelium of Mouse embryo (Hugon and Borgers, 1969), of Rat (Vollrath, 1971), of Fowl (Ono, 1973), of metamorphosing Xenopus (Bonneville and Weinstock, 1970) and of metamorphosing Insects (Van der Starre—Van der Molen and De Priester, 1972; Andries, 1972).

In our material, the microvilli of cultivated thyroid cells seem to be formed by the latter mechanism (Figs. 7—10). Numerous rounded or twisted dense vesicles, sometimes budding from the Golgi apparatus, are found in the apical cytoplasm near the follicular lumen. They contain an electron-dense material without any granular or filamentous infrastructure. Depending on the plane of section their size is about 2,000 Å in diameter and they sometimes have a double wall composed of two concentric membranes. This image might represent the cross-section of a horse-shoe shaped vesicle in a plane of section perpendicular to its axis.

During the migration of these vesicles towards the apical cell pole, their internal concave face often bears a small area where their membrane seems thicker and more electron-dense, as has been described (Vollrath, 1971) or may be recognized on micrographs from other cell species (Ono, 1973). This thickened membrane area would become the tip of the future microvillus (Fig. 10).

Many of such vesicles fuse with the apical membrane in a disordered fashion; then several microfilaments penetrate the tips, contributing to the growth of the microvilli. The dense material contained in these vesicles seems to flow into the follicular lumen after incorporation of the vesicles' membrane into the apical plasmalemma. It should be noted, however, that some images of vesicles near the apical pole might also be due to the plane of section happening to be perpendicular to the direction of development of microvilli (Fig. 10).

This phenomenon brings about a considerable increase in the apical membrane surface. The follicular lumen filled with growing microvilli and dense material brought by the Golgi vesicles is very jagged and tortuous. These changes are paralleled by formation at the apical pole of numerous coated endocytotic vesicles containing a clear material. This might represent a mechanism of at least partial membrane recovery.

4. Nature of the Dense Follicular Material

The nature of the dense material contained in the newly formed follicles could not be definitely elucidated. The following interpretations, though none of them based on conclusive evidence, can be submitted for discussion.

a) Ultimobranchial Colloid

These follicles containing osmiophilic material, instead of thyroidal, may be for instance from ultimobranchial origin. In the fresh-water Turtle the ultimo-branchial follicles are characterized by their very electron dense content (Khai-rallah and Clark, 1971) and in the Rat a small number of follicles, likely to be ultimobranchial, contain a very heterogeneous colloid (Wetzel and Wollman, 1969). But in our cultures secretion granules typical for ultimobranchial cells are absent; furthermore all the follicles observed in culture have the same appearance at the beginning of their formation, so that it is very unlikely that some of them should have a distinct origin.

b) Immature Thyroglobulin

Soon after its formation the follicular lumen can contain thyroglobulin since all the cells produce this glycoprotein, even when they are not reassociated (Tixier-Vidal, 1969; Fayet et al., 1970; Lissitzky et al., 1971). This material could then be immature thyroglobulin, e. g. imperfectly iodinated; though, as no chemical characterization of the follicular contents has been carried out we cannot assert this to be the case.

c) Thyroglobulin Modified by the Processing for Electron Microscopy

The method used for fixation can cause considerable modifications in the electron density of the contents of thyroid follicles in organotypic culture (Rose, 1970). The contents are very dense after aldehydic fixation while very weakly contrasted after osmic fixation. But this cannot explain the great density of the follicular contents for, on the one hand, all the cultures underwent double fixation by glutaraldehyde-osmium tetroxide and, on the other hand, narrow follicles with a dense content and larger follicles with a clear one can be often seen on the same grid.

In any case, it would be rash to consider the filamentous aspect observed in the microfollicles at the beginning of reassociation as significant for the presence of either immature or modified thyroglobulin. Indeed, it seems according to Berg (1974) that the thyroglobulin molecule appears to have distinctly different form and dimensions in the electron microscope. The presence of thyroglobulin in the microfollicular contents, although highly probable, is therefore not actually proved and the ultrastructural appearance does not provide any positive evidence relevant to this.

d) Cell Catabolism Products

Preliminary cytoplasmical studies, which have still to be confirmed, indicate that after 6 days of culture the dense material remaining in the follicle contains acid phosphatase, an excellent lysosomal marker enzyme. So the thyroid cells might discharge into the follicular lumen some of their waste accumulated in the cytoplasm. In any case, proteolytic activity of the colloid collected by micropuncture was already shown in the Rat (De Robertis, 1941), but this fact has been not confirmed by biochemical study of Rat colloid isolated by follicular micropuncture (Smeds, 1972).

e) Membrane Glycoproteins or "Cell Coat"

At least some of the dense material contained in the follicular lumen seems to have been brought by dense vesicles arising from the Golgi apparatus during the morphogenesis of the microvilli. During the growth of the follicle this dense material can be seen to form fine filaments which then make up a felting around the microvilli; this felting might be the glycoproteic coat of the apical plasma surface, i. e. the glycocalyx.

Many authors have studied the glycocalyx or cell coat (reviews by Cook, 1968; Martinez-Palomo, 1970; Winzler, 1970; Rambourg, 1971; Cook and Stoddart, 1973). This glycoprotein layer covers the surface of all cells and is synthetized in the Golgi apparatus, as has been shown by autoradiographic, cytochemical and biochemical studies (review: Cook, 1973).

Andries' observations (1972) seem to provide an important argument for the idea that the osmiophilic material filling the lumen of the reconstituted thyroid follicles contains the glycocalyx glycoproteins. During the metamorphosis of an Insect, Aeschna cyanea, the intestinal epithelium of the larva degenerates and then is reconstituted from small-sized cells situated near the epithelial basal lamina and without contact with the intestinal lumen. The differentiation of these cells takes place before the larval intestinal epithelium has completely desquamated and as a result of this, the basal cells grow larger between the larval intestinal cells. The new microvilli then appear enveloped in a very osmiophilic material originating from the previously described Golgi vesicles. Electron dense material containing microvilli is then situated in an enclosed space bound by the larval intestinal cells. This stage of intestinal microvilli maturation is comparable to that observed in cultured thyroid cells. Afterwards, the cell differentiates and increases in height between the larval intestinal cells, pushed aside little by little by it's apical pole, which finally reaches the intestinal lumen. At this time the dense material which is no longer contained in an enclosed space becomes diluted and spreads at the surface of the cells, apparently constituting the glycocalyx of the microvilli. The cytochemical study using Thiéry's and Rambourg's techniques seems to show that the tuft actually contains glycoproteins.

Things seem to take place in the same way in our cultures, with the difference that the dilution of the dense contents is progressive, as it can only occur during the slow enlargement of the follicle (Figs. 9–11).

5. Morphogenesis of Cilia

The presence of isolated cilia in the thyroid gland has been observed by many authors. These cilia generally protrude in the follicular cavity (Hilfer, 1964; Fujita and Tanisawa, 1966) or may occasionally be related to the lateral cell spaces (Calvert and Pusterla, 1973).

Similarly, electron microscopy revealed the presence of isolated cilia in numerous embryonic or adult cells either in vivo or cultured in vitro (review by Weathley, 1966). Isolated cilia can appear in experimentally stimulated cells (Weathley, 1967) or in epithelial cells transformed by a carcinogenic agent (Yalciner and Friedell, 1973).

These isolated cilia very often present an imperfect structure, as is the case in our cultures. The stages of their formation in cultured thyroid cells are the same as in the development of the other cells studied i. e. fibroblasts (Sorokin, 1962; Stubblefield and Brinkley, 1967) and epithelial cells of choroid plexus (Martinez-Martinez and Daems, 1968), cornea (Smith et al., 1969), trachea (Kalnins and Porter, 1969) and oviduct (McCarron and Anderson, 1973). The origin of the ciliary vesicle is still unknown. It is probably an endocytotic vesicle (Renaud and Swift, 1964) or it comes from the Golgi apparatus (Martinez-Martinez and Daems, 1969). Its appearing in vitro in the Golgi region and the analogy between the development of cilia and microvilli (according to the most currently accepted hypothesis) support the second origin.

6. Growth of the Follicle

At the beginning the early follicle is composed of only 2 or 3 epithelial cells. After several days of culture in the presence of TSH, some follicles are large in size and are made up of more than 10 cells. What are the mechanisms allowing follicle growth and the increase in the number of constituent cells ?

We never observed by light microscope examination of in situ-embedded cultures any mitoses in the follicular wall, whereas they are frequently encountered in vivo especially during the embryonic development of the gland.

It seems more likely that still isolated cells become incorporated into the epithelial wall between already reassociated cells. Some electron micrographs show extremely elongated cells with a part of their apical pole constituting but a small area of the follicular wall, while the rest of their cytoplasm almost completely envelops the other cells with which they are reassociated.

Microcinematographic studies (Fayet et al., 1971) showed the very active movements of cultured thyroid cells and clearly vizualized the fusion of follicles of varying sizes. Such fusions had already been described during the embryonic development of the thyroid gland (Norris, 1916; Hilfer, 1964).

It is not impossible that some small aggregates seen to enlarge during microcinematographic observation already possess a follicular cleft which cannot be seen in such technical condition, so that the increasing number of cells of these aggregates in fact corresponds to the incorporation of new cells into the epithelium of true already formed follicles.

It is therefore most probable that the growth of the follicular cleft requires the incorporation of new epithelial cells next to those which are already reassociated. Later, the formation of very large follicular cavities is achieved by fusion of two neighbouring cell masses. These two phenomena imply great cell motility, which is actually shown by microcinematography. This motility is probably related to the ultrastructural substrate consisting of very numerous microfilaments which can be seen in the hyaloplasm of thyroid cells in culture, as well as in many other cell types (Baker and Schroeder, 1967; Goldman and Follet, 1969; Spooner et al., 1973).

7. The Role of Hydrocortisone

The action of glycocorticoids on the metabolism of the thyroid cell is still under discussion (Yatvin et al., 1966). Hydrocortisone increases iodine uptake (Colle-van de Velde, 1969) and excretion of thyroid hormones (Colle-Van de Velde and Elewaut, 1971) by fragments of mouse fetal and perinatal thyroids cultured in vitro and stimulated by TSH.

Added at time 0 together with TSH, hydrocortisone seems to have two possibly related effects on thyroid cells in vitro. First, the biochemical approach reveals an increase in the time of survival of cells in culture together with a parallel increase in the iodine metabolism (uptake, organification) (A. Giraud, 1975). Second, the morphological approach shows an increase in size and number of lysosomal dense bodies (hydrocortisone is known to play a protective role on the lysosomal membrane: Weissman and Dingle, 1961) and the appearing of many nuclear bodies.

III. The Origin of the Follicular Lumen

We will discuss here the two currently held theories and omit discussion of the hypothesis of a tubular structure of the gland which has been abandoned long ago and still as incompatible with results of the recent study of the thyroid capillary network by Fujita and Murakami (1974) with the scanning electron microscope; the theory of cell lysis has also been discarded (cf. Introduction).

A. Hypothesis for the Formation of the Follicular Lumen from Intracytoplasmic Cavities

According to this hypothesis the follicular cavity is derived from the simultaneous fusion of several intracytoplasmic vacuoles termed microfollicular.

1. Review of the Work by Light Microscopy

This hypothesis was held by authors studying follicular morphogenesis, either in situ during embryonic life or in vitro by the light microscope, with which the early stages of follicular morphogenesis cannot be observed owing to its poor resolution.

According to our results, the follicular clefts are narrow in the beginning, measuring several microns in length but less than 0.5μ in width, and appear completely empty even of low density material.

The first colloid droplets, which appear spherical according to some authors (Knake and Riedel, 1960; Kojima, 1960; Van Heyningen, 1961; Voikevitch and Zenzerov, 1968), measure about 2 or more μ in diameter. These images, however, do not correspond to the very early stages of the formation of follicles as observed with the electron microscope, similarly to what has been previously observed by one of us in hyperactive human thyroids (Vague et al., 1968; Michel-Béchet et al., 1969; Vague et al., 1972).

2. Review of the Work in Electron Microscopy

The authors who studied follicular morphogenesis with the electron microscope have not provided a definite proof for this hypothesis.

According to Shepard (1967, 1968), the formation of the follicular lumen in the human thyroid starts with the appearance of a spherical microfollicular cavity in the cytoplasm of epithelial cells; this is about 1 μ in diameter and is bordered by microvilli. This cavity comes from the smooth endoplasmic reticulum (ER). The final follicular lumen is then formed by simultaneous fusion of several intracytoplasmic cavities situated in adjacent cells giving rise to a "clover-leaf" image. In the schema proposed by this author a very narrow canal is drawn linking the "intracytoplasmic cavity" to the intercellular space at the apical pole (cf. Plate 1 b).

These observations are open to 3 criticisms.

(1) The narrow canal drawn on the schema is not present in any of the micrographs presented by the author. If it exists, the cavity is not really intracytoplasmic since it is in continuity with the apical extracellular space.

(2) The author cannot provide any definite proof of the intracytoplasmic nature of the microfollicle, since he did not study its spatial configuration by means of serial sections in electron microscopy. Certainly, the author mentions in support of his observations the appearance and the intracytoplasmic development of these cavities as investigated in semi-thin sections of epon-embedded tissue observed with the light microscope. But the comparison of the respective sizes of the "intracytoplasmic" cavities on the semi-thin sections and corresponding electron micrographs suggests that the author may not have studied the development of the same cavity: in fact it can be admitted that the proportions between sizes of nuclei and intracytoplasmic cavities are equal in semi-thin and ultrathin sections respectively, as conditions are identical ,whereas the size of the microfollicular lumen appears on the author's illustrations at least 3 times larger in the semithin section than in the electron micrograph.

Finally, it should be noted that the hypothesis of intracytoplasmic genesis of the follicular cavity is in contradiction with the ultrastructural data concerning the differentiation of other epithelial structures (cf. Discussion, IV).

Other authors, who made similar observations of "intracytoplasmic cavities", have taken up once again Shepard's hypothesis but have neither supported it by further arguments (Garcia-Bunuel, 1972; Welsch, 1972) nor carried out the study of serial semi-thin sections (Neve and Dumont, 1970).

In 1973, Calvert and Pusterla took up the problem again by studying with te electron microscope serial sections of embryonic Rat thyroid. According to these authors, the formation of the follicle takes place through 4 stages:

(1) the first evidence of follicular organization occurs at the 17th day of pregnancy with the constitution of a circular or oval junctional complex between

two cells, measuring about 8 μ in diameter. Desmosomes are found at the periphery of this junctional complex;

(2) interdigitations of the plasmalemma then appear in the middle of the junctional complex;

(3) the microfollicular cavity, filled with microvilli, is formed at the apical pole of the cell but without relations with the apical plasma membrane bearing the interdigitations. This cavity is therefore intracytoplasmic and the authors describe small, clear vesicles between this cavity and the apical interdigitations;

(4) finally, the typical follicular lumen becomes visible a little later. It is surrounded by a circular junctional complex.

This mechanism, which is halfway between Shepard's hypothesis and that of the extracellular origin of the follicular lumen, calls for several remarks.

Firstly, to state with certainty that the first step of follicular organization is the formation of a disc-shaped zone of cell contact where the plasma membranes fuse to form a zonula occludens surrounded by desmosomes, the authors must have examined serial sections through a tissue slice at least 8 μ thick corresponding to the diameter of this zone. Furthermore, to exclude the existence of any follicular cavity situated outside this zone the total thickness examined should be still greater. Assuming that each section is about 800 Å thick and that the plane of section is approximately perpendicular to the plane containing the cell junction, the authors should have examined about 100 consecutive sections. Their conclusions would be more convincing had their results been substantiated by detailed numerical tables showing that such a serial observation had been done.

Secondly assuming that the follicular cavity appears in the center of a disc-shaped zone of cell junction, the zonula occludens where the external sheets of the plasmalemmas are fused has a circular spatial configuration and must be surrounded by the zonula adherens and desmosomes; consequently the zone of circular junction sectioned along its greatest diameter is symmetrical respecting its center. Thus from one extremity of the section to the other we must necessarily see the succession of an intercellular space, a desmosome (which can be missing), a zonula adherens, the zonula occludens, a second zonula adherens, another desmosome (which may be absent in the section examined) and finally the intercellular space of the opposite pole. In the electron micrograph presented by the authors, however, this zone of junction is asymmetrical since it presents the succession of the 3 elements making up a single junctional complex: a zonula occludens, a zonula adherens and a desmosome.

Thirdly, the question arises as to what happens to the interdigitations in the center of this zone of junction when the "intracytoplasmic" cavities fuse to give rise to the follicular lumen and whether they have any relation with microvilli.

Lastly, this interpretation disagrees with the subsequent work published by the same group (Calvert, 1973), on alkaline phosphatase activity during the embryonic development of the Rat thyroid. At the 15th day of gestation the epithelial cells, disposed in clusters, contain no cavity interpretable as an intracytoplasmic follicular lumen. After the 16th day of gestation, the small follicular lumina containing microvilli only appear between 2 or 3 cells. High power view of the apical pole of these cells reveals that two types of structures display an alkaline phosphatase activity: one is the content of the Golgi saccules and the inside surface of the membranes of the small, clear vesicles about 1,000 Å in diameter which seem to fuse with the apical membrane; the other type consists of the external face of the membranes of the microvilli and follicular plasmalemma. At this stage, the lateral faces of the cells lack a detectable enzymatic activity. These observations on the one hand confirm the hypothesis proposed for the morphogenesis of the microvilli and show, on the other hand, that the cell junctions described on the 17th day as the first stage of folliculogenesis are in fact late stages when the follicles are already formed.

The same conclusions can be drawn from the study of the appearance of peroxidase during the development of the Rat embryonic thyroid (Strum et al., 1973).

In conclusion, the hypothesis of the formation of the follicular lumen from "intracytoplasmic cavities" does not seem to be supported by indisputable observations. If it were the case, the thyroid follicle cell would be an exception among epithelial cells (we will come back to this point) and, furthermore, the observations we made in our cultures seem to invalidate such a hypothesis.

It should be noted that it was proposed by authors studying the embryonic morphogenesis of the gland in situ. However, the great disadvantage of using embryonic material is the uncertain determination of its exact age especially in the higher Vertebrates where it cannot be determined with great accuracy.

Thus it is often difficult to state with certainty the exact sequence of structural organizations representing successive developmental events. Shepard, on the one hand, and Calvert and Pustela, on the other hand, consider as the first stage cells possessing microvilli and extremely developed (8 µ) cell junctions, while most authors and even Calvert himself, have shown the existence of an early stage of development where the epithelial cells possess neither a means of union nor microvilli. So it should be pointed to some unavoidable uncertainty of interpretations based solely on such material.

B. Hypothesis of the Formation of the Follicular Lumen from the Intercellular Space Partitioned by an Annular Zonula Occludens

The study of reassociation of isolated adult thyroid cells in culture confirms the work of those authors and in particular Hilfer (1964, 1968) who have analysed the development of the gland or what happens to embryonic thyroid cells in culture.

1. Review of the Literature

The Stages of Follicular Reassociation in Vitro

Observations of the stages in thyroid follicle formation is difficult with the light microscope. Nevertheless, several authors described long ago images of colloid secretion in triangular-shaped spaces between epithelial cells.

This triangular form of follicle seen by the light microscope probably corresponds to the clover-leaf electron microscope images described or shown by many authors (Feldman et al., 1961; Hajos et al., 1964; Hilfer, 1964; Fujita and Tanisawa, 1966). Such images are interpreted by those investigators favouring the theory of intracytoplasmic formation as the stage of fusion of microfollicular cavities. These clover-leaf images were also seen in our cultures (Fig. 13b, p. 13 and Fig. 14b, p. 28) and could be due to two concomitant phenomena.

Firstly, the considerable increase in the membrane surface caused by the appearance of microvilli leads to invagination of apical cell pole. This mechanism was described in the human embryonic thyroid gland (Lietz et al., 1971).

Secondly, it can be supposed that the growth of the junctional complex is slower than the increase in the apical surface or that the means of cell union are more rigid than the other parts of the plasma membrane.

The disproportionate evolution between the increase in the plasma membrane and the growth of the junctional complex could explain the numerous cloverleaf or daisy-like images seen in certain stages of follicular development. This phenomenon was already observed during development of fowl embryonic thyroid (Hilfer, 1964).

It should be noted that these images do not represent the initial stages of follicular development but rather already advanced stages the appearance of the microvilli when the follicular volume has become large enough. The apical pole of the epithelial cells takes the shape of hemispherical domes of various diameters situated between the junctional complexes. The cross-section of the follicular lumen is therefore never a circle or perfect oval but has an irregular outline composed of a series of scallops of unequal radii joined together at their extremities by junctional complexes.

The authors describe during the embryonic development of the gland in vivo (Feldman et al., 1961; Hajos et al., 1964; Ishikawa, 1965; Fujita and Tanizawa, 1966) or during the differentiation in vitro of the explanted embryonic gland (Petrovic and Porte, 1961; Daems and Thesing, 1962; Hilfer et al., 1968; Spooner, 1970) a stage in which the juxtaposed epithelial elements in the early follicle lack any differentiated cell junction. This was also the case in our culture (Fig. 4). This stage is common to all epithelial cells during their differentiation.

The reassociation of isolated embryonic cells is very rapid since a follicular cleft is formed at about the 8th h of culture (Hilfer and Hilfer, 1966). The very narrow early form of the follicle appears between two cells (Hilfer, 1968) or several cells (Feldman et al., 1961) and in this case is very irregularly shaped. Though initially sparse, the microvilli eventually fill up almost completely the still very narrow lumen which consequently cannot be distinguished by the light microscope. Hilfer (1964) shows in micrographs and graphically in a schema two distinct follicular cavities between three associated cells. Thus one cell could possess two different apical poles bordering two distinct follicular lumina (Fig. 1a). This would seem little likely and it is more probable that these images are due to two sections in the same plane of section of a single, tortuous follicular cavity stretching between several thyroid cells.

The numerous images of narrow follicular clefts provide convincing evidence for the extracellular origin of the follicle and tend to disparage the hypothesis of fusion of intracytoplasmic cavities.

2. Proofs Supporting this Hypothesis

Two types of supplementary evidence substantiate the conclusion of the last paragraph namely a) the study of ultrathin serial sections and b) the construction and examination of sections obtained from a follicular model.

a) The Study of Ultrathin Serial Sections

By systematically examining sections collected on 3 grids from each block of 4–6 day-old cultures, we found on two occasions in two serial sections not far from each other, an image weakening Shepard's theory of the "intracytoplasmic microfollicular cavity". Firstly, 3 thus defined cavities lie side by side in three neighbouring cells (Fig. 13a, p. 26; Fig. 14a, p. 28). However, in several sections further along these cavities fuse together to give rise to the characteristic clover-leaf image (Fig. 13b, 14b). This phenomenon is found in small-sized cavities comparable to those described by Shepard (Fig. 13) as well as in larger-sized cavities (Fig. 14).

The serial sections of early (4–6 days) cultures of thyroid cells demonstrate that the "intracytoplasmic cavities" seen are, in fact, tangential sections of "clover-leaf" follicles. Two series of micrographs (Figs. 13 and 14) do not constitute sufficient proof to formally refute Shepard's hypothesis. Though they show that the "intracytoplasmic cavities" may result from improper interpretation, they do not contribute any data on the mechanism of formation of the clover-leaf follicular cavity. Furthermore, the sections were obtained from 4 or more day-old cultures and so we cannot discard the possibility that the formation of the follicular lumen did not take place before three days in culture by the mechanism described by Shepard.

We therefore examined serial sections of very short-term cultures (3 h and 12 h) in two planes, respectively parallel and perpendicular to the surface of the culture through a thickness of around 10 μ. At this stage all the follicular lumina examined are narrow clefts bordered by microvilli and contain electron-dense material. Several cavities which might be "intracytoplasmic" are found, especially in the sections perpendicular to the culture, but they are due to the sinuous contours of the extracellular follicular lumen.

b) Study of Follicular Models (Fig. 15, p. 29)

Using plasticine models that can be cut in many different planes, it is possible to easily explain that the "intracytoplasmic" images in fact only represent particular incidences of section of more or less large, branched follicular cavities.

When the follicular lumen with or without a border of microvilli is very narrow, all the planes of section reveal a very elongated cavity at the extremities of which exist an adult junctional complex or an isolated zonula occludens. It is very difficult in this case to obtain intracytoplasmic, microfollicular cavity images. This confirms the results obtained from the study of serial sections of early cultures (3–12 h).

When the follicle is larger in size and is composed of 3 or 4 epithelial cells the images seen in a cell can be classified into 3 principal types depending on whether the plane of section is more or less tangential or oblique in respect to a fictive sphere, the center of which is in the middle of the follicular lumen. The three types are as follows:

(1) if the plane of section is very close to the center or passes through the center of this sphere, the clover-leaf image is obtained (Fig. 15: plane of section A; compare with Figs. 13b, 14b);

(2) if the plane of section does not pass through the center of the follicle and is oblique, the image obtained is one of an "intracytoplasmic microfollicular cavity" not far from which is found a junctional complex, more of less complete because it is sectionned by a tangential plane (Fig. 15: plane of section B; compare with Fig. 10);

(3) finally, in a very tangential section the junctional complex disappears and is replaced by the lateral face of the cell and its finger-like extensions (Fig. 15: plane of section C; compare with Figs. 11a, 13a).

48

These three types of different images can be seen by sectioning the same follicular cavity in the various cells which make up the follicular wall. For example, in Fig. 14a, a cavity sectioned according to plane B can be seen as well as two cavities sectioned in plane A.

The results of the study of the time course of reassociation of isolated thyroid cells together with the examination of serial ultrathin sections and the study of models provide evidence against the hypothesis of formation of the follicular lumen by the fusion of intracytoplasmic microfollicular cavities. This lumen is in fact derived from the intercellular space separating the reassociated cells.

IV. Comparative Arguments Supporting the Extracellular Origin of the Follicular Lumen

This hypothesis is supported by two series of facts emerging 1—from the study of the thyroid phylogenic development and 2—from consideration of the differentiation of epithelial cells among which several examples have been chosen.

A. Phylogenic Development of the Thyroid Gland

The thyroid gland which appears in the phylum for the first time at the time of metamorphosis of the Lamprey larva is derived from the endostyle (or hypobranchial gland or subpharyngeal gland) situated in the cephalic part of the larva (Kraentzel, 1933; Leach, 1939; Clements-Merlini, 1960; Constantinescu, 1972; Suzuki and Kondo, 1973).

1. Formation and Histology of the Lamprey Endostyle (Subpharyngeal Gland)

The endostyle develops at the expense of the cephalic pharyngeal floor in the form of a groove which takes on a tubular form lying horizontally under the pharynx.

Little by little this tube becomes isolated from the pharyngeal lumen by the formation of folds of connective tissue which push the anterior wall to the back and the posterior wall forward. The endostyle communicates only with the pharyngeal lumen at its median part by a small vertical tube.

A connective tissue partition then divides the anterior part of the endostyle into two horizontal tubes parallel to the pharynx which remain connected in the median zone of the hypobranchial pouch at the point where the vertical tube communicates with the pharyngeal lumen. An identical but incomplete partition is formed in the posterior part which folds back on itself during the elongation of the endostyle.

This organ is covered by a cylindrical epithelium composed of several types of cells arranged in bands parallel to the antero-posterior axis of the larva. In particular, two types of cells, ciliated and glandular, the exact nature of the secretion products of which has not yet been elucidated. Radioautography shows that some cells take up iodine.

2. Appearance of the Thyroid Gland

At the time of larval metamorphosis cell death occurs resulting in total isolation of the subpharyngeal gland from the pharyngeal cavity. Part of the epithelial wall of the endostyle disappears and the remaining ciliated and glandular cells form typical thyroid follicles by radial reorganization around a lumen derived from the endostylic cavity.

The phylogenic development of the thyroid gland therefore furnishes interesting arguments for the theory of extracellular follicle formation, since the follicular lumen derives from the endostylic cavity in Ammocoete larvae.

Two further remarks should be made:

firstly, the evolution of the endostyle is, in fact, that of the progressive transformation of an exocrine gland (the secretory products of which might play a role in the digestive processes) into an endocrine gland. The Ammocoete constitutes a turning point in this evolution;

secondly, the presence of imperfect cilia in the cultures of thyroid cells might represent a phylogenic remnant of the cilia of endostylic epithelium (Fujita, 1963).

B. General Cytologic Aspects of Differentiation of Epithelia

1. Data Relevant to the Problem

The thyroid cell is an epithelial cell derived from the floor of the primordial pharynx. The mechanisms by which this cell acquires the morphology and functional activity characteristic of the adult state are identical to those described in numerous other types of epithelial cells.

The simplest way of tackling the problem of the formation of the thyroid follicle during embryonic life is to study the differentiation of a simple epithelial cell rather than investigating the appearance of an intracytoplasmic or extracellular cavity. The problem then consists of studying three phenomena:

(1) the creation and maturation of junctions between several epithelial cells which is the initial stage in the acquisition of the morphological characteristics specific of the differentiated cell;

(2) the appearance and development of microvilli which are the morphological sign of a particular functional activity;

(3) production and secretion by the cell of molecules which are the major expression of its specific differentiation.

These three phenomena allow us to define the adult thyroid follicle as an enclosed cavity bounded by two or several epithelial cells joined together by a junctional complex bordered by microvilli which ruffle the apical poles. This cavity is filled with colloid secreted by the follicular cells.

This approach led us to search for recently published (since 1960) and mainly ultrastructural data concerning these 3 phenomena. These were obtained from studies of the embryonic development of tissues and organs or of the fate of tissues or organs either cultured in vitro or grafted in vivo. It concords both with our results and the theory of the extracellular origin of the follicular lumen.

2. Reaggregation of Dissociated Embryonic Cells

In vitro reaggregation of isolated cells of Urchin (Millonig and Giudice, 1967; Timourian et al., 1973), Triton (Feldman, 1955), Fowl (Overton, 1962) and Mouse (Stern, 1972) blastulae takes place through two successive steps.

First of all, the cell junctions which are seen with the electron microscope to be of the zonula occludens or the desmosome type are reconstituted. Then the cells form a blastula if the embryos are very young, or neural or enteric tubes if the embryos are older. According to most authors the blastocoele and tubes arise from the radial rearrangement of the cells delimiting them. As for the thyroid gland, the hypothesis of confluence of intracytoplasmic microcavities has been proposed (Millonig and Giudice, 1967), but no morphological evidence has been furnished. Cell junctions are indispensable for the acquisition of morphological biochemical features of differentiated cells. As we observed in our cultures, no morpho-functional maturation is seen in the cells that remain isolated.

The same sequence has been described during the reaggregation of embryonic cells obtained from Chick embryo neuroretina. In this case, all the authors (Sheffield and Moscona, 1969, 1970; Fujisawa, 1973; Adler, 1973) admit that the lumen of the neural tube arises from the space between the apical poles of the reaggregated cells.

3. Development of the Blood Capillaries

Again the same pattern of development is observed in the capillary network of the cerebral cortex in the fetal (Bär and Wolff, 1972) and newborn Rat (Caley and Maxwell, 1970) and of the spinal cord (Phelps, 1972), as well as during morphogenesis of the blood capillaries in tissue fragments cultured in diffusion chambers and implanted in the peritoneum (Aloisi and Schiaffino, 1971). Thus zonulae occludentes appear at contacts between undifferentiated cells which thereby delimit an almost virtual space, so that these joined cells make up the endothelial wall. The early capillary lumen is very narrow and sinuous and gradually enlarges, while a basal lamina separates the endothelial elements from the surrounding tissue.

4. Morphogenesis of Kidney Glomeruli and Tubules

The morphogenesis of the kidney glomeruli and tubules during embryonic life (Jokelainen, 1963; Osathanondh and Potter, 1966; Vetter and Gibley, 1966) and in vitro (Saxen and Wartiowaara, 1966; Wartiowaara, 1966a and b) occurs in a similar way as in thyroid follicles in vivo and in vitro. There is in fact a very close analogy between the developing embryonic kidney glomerulus and the thyroid follicle. The early glomerulus consists of a cluster of several cells which join together to form a spherule totally isolated from the tubular segments of the nephron. The lumen of this early glomerulus is at first very narrow since the apical poles of cells which constitute it are closely facing each other. After it has acquired its spherical form by radial rearrangement of the cells, the glomerular lumen enlarges before being flattened by the growth of the bud of vascular connective tissue which will constitute the flocculus. The continuity between the future glomerular urinary chamber and the lumen of the proximal segment of the nephron is established secondarily.

5. Organogenesis and Histogenesis of the Pancreas

Ultrastructural studies of organogenesis and histogenesis of the pancreas also weaken the theory of the intracellular origin of ducts or acini. The primordial pancreas, which arises from an evagination of the intestinal wall, appears pseudostratified with the light microscope. However, by electron microscopy, it can be seen that the epithelial cells in fact form a unistratified epithelium, are joined together by zonulae occludentes, and possess several microvilli which protrude into the very narrow and twisted lumen of the duct. The only difference from the embryonic thyroid gland is that the primitive pancreatic cells very early have microvilli. Though, it should be kept in mind that these cells are derived from the intestinal epithelium which also possesses microvilli at the same stage (Pictet et al., 1972).

6. Morphogenesis of the Biliary Canaliculi of the Liver Parenchyme

Morphogenesis of the biliary canaliculi in the liver also takes place in the same way. During the embryonic development of the Chick (Karrer and Cox, 1962; Jones, 1963; Franceschini and Motta, 1970), Mouse (Peters et al., 1963; Wilson, 1963), Rat (Dadoune, 1963; Dvorak, 1964; Wood, 1965; de Wolf-Peeters et al., 1972), Man (Zamboni, 1965), and during the postnatal growth of the Rabbit (Carruthers and Steiner, 1962) and the Rat (Dvorak and Mazanec, 1967), the biliary canaliculi appear between two hepatocytes or between the triangle formed by three hepatic cells. The cell junctions are zonulae occludentes with sometimes a desmosome. The immature biliary canaliculi only have a few microvilli which increase at a later stage.

All authors who have studied this problem agree that the "intracytoplasmic" biliary canaliculi described in the early stages of hepatocyte differentiation in Carassius auratus (David, 1961) or in the human embryo (Koga, 1971) are only the consequence of particular incidences of section and that they do not really exist. This fact, already established by histochemical studies (Novikoff and Noe, 1955), has been recently confirmed by studies of embryonic Rat liver cells in culture (Lambiotte et al., 1972). It was found that hepatocytes isolated from fetal glands by trypsinization and culture in vitro, under the influence of hydrocortisone reconstitute biliary canaliculi from interstices separating the cells. The maturation of these biliary canaliculi is similar to that observed in situ. The effect of hydro-cortisone is reversible.

Once again the Lamprey seems to be the ideal material to confirm this me-chanism as accounting for the genesis of the biliary canaliculus. According to De Vos et al. (1973), the liver of the Lamprey larva is a tubular gland, the cells of which are organized around the primordial bile ducts. The liver of Myxine glutinosa is also tubular according to Mugnaini and Harboe (1967), but con-clusions of these authors are at variance with results of Elias and Bengelsdorf (1952).

7. Development of Gastric Oxyntic Cells

The study of the oxyntic cells present in the lining of gastric fundic glands also provides interesting data. These hydrochloric acid secreting cells present two different morphological appearances in Amphibians and higher Vertebrates especially Mammals.

In Amphibians, the oxyntic cells appear during metamorphosis and hydro-chloric acid secretion starts parallelly with their cytological differentiation (Forte et al., 1969). The undifferentiated cells are cubical and have no apical microvilli; their cytoplasm contains large amounts of free ribosomes and only few smooth ER cavities. After metamorphosis, the cell modifications are considerable. Microvilli appear at the apical cell pole and the ER increases considerably. The starting of HCL secretion by ingestion of food or by the action of specific pharma-cological agents (histamin, gastrin) allows observation of a slight increase in the surface of the apical plasmalemma and of images of openings in the ER cisternae at the base of the microvilli. This candicular system very probably plays a role in HCL secretion (Vial and Orrego, 1960; Sedar, 1961, 1969a, b).

In Mammals, the embryonic oxyntic cells are comparable to those of Amphibians before metamorphosis. Their differentiation does not result in considerable development of the ER, but in the appearance of so-called "intracellular canaliculi" studded with microvilli and widely open at the apical pole of the cells. These canaliculi, which had formerly been demonstrated by silver impregnation technique (Zimmerman, 1898), are derived from very deep invaginations in the cytoplasm of the apical plasmalemma with its microvilli, as has been described in the human (Nomura, 1966), Rabbit (Hayward, 1967) and Rat (Helander, 1969) embryos. Food ingestion and specific stimulation of HCL secretion bring about modifications which are comparable with those described in Amphibians.

These observations are extremely interesting since they indicate the close relationships existing between the smooth ER and the apical plasmalemma bearing the microvilli. They show that in both classes of Vertebrates there is a sort of balance between the development of the smooth reticulum and that of the so-called "intracytoplasmic canaliculi". In Amphibians the oxyntic cells, the ER of which is very developed, do not have such canaliculi lined with microvilli. In Mammals, on the contrary, the canaliculi become considerably developed by invagination of the apical plasmalemma while the smooth ER is reduced. In both cases, the only relationship existing between these two membrane systems are temporary openings of the ER cisternae at the apical poles. A comparison can be drawn between this process and that of thyroid folliculogenesis since once again cavities related to secretory activity are seen to be formed not from the ER, but from extensions of extracellular spaces, the widening of which pushes apart and flattens apical cell poles.

8. Conclusion

The study of cell maturation in covering or glandular epithelia during their embryonic development or in cultures in vitro allows to draw attention on several general developmental features applying to various epithelial cells and in particular to thyroid cells.

(1) At a very early stage of their development the cells form small clusters without any differentiated cell junction. Their plasma membrane is devoid of microvilli.

(2) Morphological and functional differentiation of the cells requires the establishment of cell junctions at first consisting of a zonula occludens to which can be later added a zonula adherens and one or several desmosomes.

(3) The formation of these cell junctions confers a polarity on the epithelial cells allowing them to delimit a cavity which is at first very narrow and branched, and which then becomes more or less spherical by radial rearrangement of the cells making up the wall.

(4) Microvilli, the number of which varies according to the cell type under consideration, spring up from the apical pole of the cells, which was formerly devoid of any extension.

These four stages are common to the differentiation of most normal epithelial cells. It even seems that pathological cells, particularly in thyroid, keep this pattern of organization and relations with the neighbouring cells of the same type:

small follicular cavities bound by a small number of epithelial cells have been described in toxic thyroid nodules (Michel-Béchet et al., 1968), in goitres (Heiman, 1966), in thyroids of the Quervain's thyroiditis (Volpe et al., 1967; Neve, 1970; Bastenie et al., 1972), as well as in some types of thyroid carcinoma. Similar structures have also been seen in epithelial tumors from tissues as different as the kidney (Cooper and Waisman, 1973) and the ependymal epithelium (Luse, 1960; Escola-Pico, 1963; Hirano and Zimmerman, 1967; Poon et al., 1971; Goebel and Craviotti, 1972).

Summary

Porcine thyroid cells, isolated by trypsinization from adult glands and cultured in vitro in a medium containing thyrotropin (TSH), begin to reassociate within 15 min and, within a week, or more when hydrocortisone is added to TSH, regain their previous in vivo follicular organization. Cells cultured without TSH-stimulation behave similarly, though transiently during only the first days of culture. After about four days a monolayer culture extend over the surface of the plastic support. The TSH-stimulated cells also lose their three-dimensional organization after more than a week.

The morphogenesis of the thyroid follicles was observed with the electron microscope from time 0 (end of cell isolation and beginning of culture) until the 11th day.

Particular attention was paid to short term cultures, which allowed us to observe that the follicular lumen originates from a part of the space between 2 or more epithelial cells. This space is isolated by reconstitution of a cell junction, which at this stage is a zonula occludens. Observation of serial ultrathin sections and follicular models supports this statement.

About the 12th h, the early thyroid follicle is filled with numerous intermingled microvilli and an intervillous electron dense material made of heterogeneous components. At this stage, it is likely to contain immature or mature thyroid colloid, a glycoproteic material probably related to the glycocalyx of the apical surface of epithelial cells and their microvilli, and perhaps also residues of cell catabolism.

After several days, the follicle grows in two ways: first by incorporation of still non-reassociated cells and later through fusion of neighbouring follicles. The large follicles appear in section as composed of five or more cells surrounding a colloid of the same electron density as in gland follicles in vivo submitted to identical fixation and staining processing.

This mechanism of follicular lumen formation originating from the inter-cellular space appears in this case to result from reciprocal behaviour common to a great number of epithelial cells. Epithelial cells from various embryonic adult or neoplastic tissues, either in vitro or in vivo, isolate a part of the intercellular space, first by a zonula occludens, then by a more elaborate junctional complex, and form canalicular, tubular or vesicular structures in the same way as do thyroid cells in the present study. This similarity is illustrated by some examples recently documented in the literature.

This aspect of follicular morphogenesis has been previously described by authors studying either the embryologic development of the thyroid, or the behaviour of dissociated cells grafted in vivo or cultured in vitro, or comparative aspects of the thyroid in phylogenic evolution. Therefore, it seems that the adult thyroid cells, in such conditions as in vitro culture following isolation by trypsinization appear similar to embryonic thyroid cells.

Besides, as seems to be the case during the embryologic development of the thyroid gland, thyrotropin, though necessary for the maintenance and growth of reconstituted new follicles, does not seem to play any important role during the first steps of the follicular morphogenesis in culture.

In conclusion, thyroid morphogenesis as it occurred in our experimental conditions agreed rather well the dual functional behaviour of the gland. The first, common to all endocrine glands, is the secretion into the blood stream of thyroid hormones from the basal pole of follicular cells, and the second is very similar to that of an exocrine gland. This view si supported by the fact that the thyroid epithelium is an exocrine and probably digestive gland during early stages of its phylogenic evolution, i. e. before the metamorphosis of Ammocoetes; thereafter, though the thyroid gland secretes and accumulates colloid in a closed pseudo-acinar cavity, the fundamental dynamic processes of exocrine epithelial tissue organization are maintained.

Acknowledgements

We wish to thank Prof. D. Picard for his supervision of this work and Prof. S. Lissitzky for pertinent advice. We thank also the staff of the Medical Biochemistry Laboratory for the tissue cultures and discussion of the results namely Misses S. Hovsepian, H. Damais, O. Guiringhelli, A. Giraud, Drs. J. Mauchamp, R. Planells and Mr. B. Verrier. The invaluable assistance of Mrs. A. M. Athouël-Haon and Mr. C. Cataldo in photography and electron microscopy and Mrs. J. Bottini in preparing the manuscript is also acknowledged. We wish to thank Mrs. C. Lipcey and Mr. A. Lipcey for translation of french text.

References

Adler, R.: Cell interactions and histogenesis in embryonic neural aggregates. Expt. Cell Res. **77**, 367–375 (1973)

Almquist, S., Olin, P., Ekholm, R.: La biosynthèse de la thyroglobuline en liaison avec l'ultrastructure de la thyroide foetale humaine et l'apparition de thyréotrophine immuno-réactive dans la glande pituitaire du foetus. p. 31. Fellinger, F. et Hofer, R., Eds. VIth International Thyroid Conference, Vienna 1970

Aloisi, M., Schiaffino, S.: Growth of elementary blood vessels in diffusion chambers. II. Electron microscopy of capillary morphogenesis. Virchows Arch. Abt. B 8, 328–341 (1971)

Andries, J. C.: Genèse intraépithéliale des microvillosités de l'épithélium mésentérique de la larve d'Aeschna cyanea. J. Microsc. Paris 15, 181–204 (1972)

Arzania, R., Larsen, W. J., Loewenstein, W. R.: The membrane junctions in communicating cells, their hybrids and segregants. Proc. nat. Acad. Sci. (Wash.) 71, 880–884 (1974)

Baker, P. C., Schroeder, T. E.: Cytoplasmic filaments and morphogenetic movement in the Amphibian neural tube. Develop. Biol. 15, 432–450 (1967)

Baker, T. G., Young, B. A.: Organ culture of the Rat thyroid gland. Experientia (Basel) **29**, 1548–1550 (1973)

Balsamo, J., Lilien, J.: Embryonic cell aggregation: kinetics and specificity of binding of enhancing factors. Proc. nat. Acad. Sci. (Wash.) 71, 727–731 (1974)

Bär, T., Wolf, J. R.: The formation of capillary basement membranes during internal vascularization of the Rat's cerebral cortex. Z. Zellforsch. **133**, 231–248 (1972)

Bargmann, W.: Histologie und mikroskopische Anatomie des Menschen: Die Schilddrüse. p. 347. Stuttgart: G. Thieme 1956

Barkley, D. S.: Adenosine-3', 5' phosphate: identification as acrasin in a species of cellular slime mold. Science **165**, 1133–1135 (1969)

Bearn, J. G.: The role of the foetal pituitary in the development and the growth of the foetal thyroid. J. Endocr. **32**, 213–214 (1966)

Berg, G.: An electron microscopic study of the thyroglobulin molecule. J. Ultrastruct. Res. **42**, 324–336 (1974)

Beug, H., Katz, F. F., Gerisch, G.: Dynamics of antigenic membrane sites relating to cell aggregation in Dictyostelium discoideum. J. Cell Biol. **56**, 647–658 (1973)

Biedl, A.: Innere Sekretion. Ihre physiologischen Grundlagen und ihre Bedeutung für die Pathologie. Histologie der Schilddrüse, 2. Aufl., Teil 1, p. 39–43. Berlin: Urban & Schwarzenberg 1913. Cited by Sugiyama, 1971

Blümcke, S., Niedorf, H. R., Rode, J., Kudszus, G.: Feinstrukturelle Veränderungen des Cornea-epithels in der Gewebekultur. III. Die Desmosomen. Z. Zellforsch. **84**, 189–198 (1968)

Boeynaems, J. M., Goldstein-Golaire, J., Dumont, J. E.: Non inactivation of TSH by Dog thyroid tissue in vitro. Endocrinology **93**, 1227–1229 (1973)

Bonner, J. T., Hall, E. M., Noller, J., Oleson, F. B., Roberts, A. B.: Synthesis of cyclic AMP and phosphodiesterase in various species of cellular slime molds and its bearing on chemotaxis and differentiation. Develop. Biol. **29**, 402–409 (1972)

Bonnet, R.: Grundriß der Entwicklungsgeschichte der Haussäugetiere. p. 138–139. Berlin: P. Parey 1891

Bonneville, M. A., Weinstock, M.: Brush border development in the intestinal absorptive cells of Xenopus during metamorphosis. J. Cell Biol. **44**, 151–171 (1970)

Booyse, F. M., Rafelson, M. E.: Regulation and mechanism of platelet aggregation. Ann. N.Y. Acad. Sci. **201**, 37–60 (1972)

Borysenko, J. Z., Revel, J. P.: Experimental manipulation of desmosome structure. Amer. J. Anat. **137**, 403–422 (1973)

Boyd, J. D.: Development of the human thyroid gland. In: The thyroid gland (Pitt-Rivers R. & Trotter W. R., Eds.) p. 9–31. Washington: Butterworth 1964

Bradway, W.: The morphogenesis of the thyroid follicles of the Chick. Anat. Rec. **42**, 157–167 (1929)

Broman, J.: Entwicklung der Schilddrüse in normaler und abnormaler Entwicklung des Menschen. p. 288–289. München: J. F. Bermann 1911. Cited by Norris 1916, Taxi 1959

Bucciante, L., Maspes, P. E.: Sulla morfogenesi della ghiandola tiroide nell'uomo e in altri mammiferi. Arch. ital. Anat. Embriol. **27**, 419–465 (1930)

Burke, G., Szabo, M.: Effects of thyroglobulin on thyroid function. J. clin. Endocr. **35**, 552–560 (1972)

Caley, D. W., Maxwell, D. S.: Development of the blood vessels and extracellular spaces during postnatal maturation of Rat cerebral cortex. J. Comp. Neurol. **138**, 31–48 (1970)

Calvert, R.: Ultrastructural localization of alkaline phosphatase activity in the developing thyroid gland of the Rat. Anat. Rec. **177**, 359–375 (1973)

Calvert, R., Pusterla, A.: Formation of thyroid follicular lumina in Rat embryo studied with serial fine sections. Gen. comp. Endocr. **20**, 584–587 (1973)

Carpenter, E., Rondon-Tarchetti, T.: Differentiation of embryonic Rat thyroid in vivo and in vitro. J. Exp. Zool. **136**, 393–417 (1958)

Carrel, A., Burrows, M. T.: Cultures primaires, secondaires et tertiaires de glande thyroïde et culture de péritoine. C. R. Soc. Biol. (Paris) **2**, 328–331 (1910)

Carrel, A., Burrows, M. T.: Cultivation of adult tissues and organs outside of the body. J. Amer. med. Assoc. **55**, 1379–1381 (1910)

McCarron, L. K., Anderson, E.: A cytological study of the postnatal development of the Rabbit oviduct epithelium. Biol. Reproduction **8**, 11–28 (1973)

Carruthers, J. S., Steiner, J. W.: Fine structure of terminal branches of the biliary tree. III. Parenchymal cell cohesion and "intracellular bile canaliculi". Arch. Pathol. **74**, 117–126 (1962)

Cauldwell, C. B., Henkart, P., Humphreys, T.: Physical properties of Sponge aggregation factor. A unique proteoglycan complex. Biochemistry (Wash.) **12**, 3051–3055 (1973)

Champy, C.: Résultats de la méthode de culture des tissus en dehors de l'organisme. Presse méd. **22**, 87–89 (1914)

Champy, C.: Quelques résultats de la méthode des cultures de tissus. V. La Glande thyroïde. Arch. Zool. Exp. Gén. **55**, 61–79 (1915)

Chardard-Raimbault, S.: Etude histochemique de la localisation de la phosphatase alcaline dans la thyroïde embryonnaire de Souris au cours de son développement et de son entrée en fonction. Arch. Anat. micr. Morph. exp. ,**42**, 102–111 (1953)

Chernly, C., Mu, J.: Thyrotropin-like activity of thyroid RNA in vitro. Proc. Soc. Exp. Biol. Med. **142**, 600–603 (1973)

Clements-Merlini, M.: The secretory cycle of iodoproteins in Ammocoetes: 2-A radioautographic study of the transforming larval thyroid gland. J. Morphol. **106**, 357–364 (1960)

Cohen, M. H., Robertson, A.: Chemotaxis and the early stages of aggregation in cellular slime molds. J. theor. Biol. **31**, 119–130 (1971)

Colle-Van de Velde, A.: Influence de l'hydrocortisone sur les thyroides foetales et périnatales de Souris, cultivées in vitro. C. R. Acad. Sci. **268**, Sér. D., 3187–3188 (1969)

Colle-Van de Velde, A., Elewant, A.: Sécrétion hormonale in vitro par dos fragments thyroïdiens de Souris: influence de l'hydrocortisone. C. R. Acad. Sci. **273** Sér. D, 3187–3188 (1969)

Constantinescu, E.: Phylogeny of the thyroid gland. Rev. Roum. Embryol. Cytol. **9**, 205–232 (1972)

Cook, G. M. W.: Glycoproteins in membranes. Biol. Rev. **43**, 363–391 (1968)

Cook, G. M. W.: The Golgi apparatus, form and function. 3. The involvement of the Golgi apparatus in the biosynthesis of glycoproteins. In: Lysosomes in biology and pathology (J. T. Dingle, Ed.) .Vol. 3, p. 256–258. Amsterdam: North Holland Publ. Cy 1973

Cook, G. M. W., Stoddart, R. W.: Surface carbohydrates of the eukaryotic cell London: Acad. Press 1973

Cooper, E. R. A.: The histology of the more important human endocrine organs at various ages. The thyroid gland. p. 56–76. London: Oxford Univ. Press 1925. Cited by Sugiyama, 1971

Cooper, P., Waisman, J.: Tubular differentiation and basement membrane production in a renal adenoma: ultrastructural features. J. Pathol. **109**, 113–122 (1973)

Curtiss, A. S. G.: Cell contact and adhesion. Biol. Rev. **37**, 82–129 (1962)

Daday, H.: The mechanism of aggregation of neural retina cells in vitro. Wilhelm Roux' Archives **171**, 244–255 (1972)

Dadoune, J. P.: Contribution à l'étude au microscope électronique de la différenciation de la cellule hépatique chez le Rat. Arch. Anat. micr. Morphol. exp. **52**, 513–571 (1963)

Daems, W. T., Thesingh, C. W.: Electron microscopy of TSH-stimulated embryonic Chick thyroids. In: Electron Microscopy (5th Intern. Congr. for Electron Microscopy, Philadelphia 1962) (Breese, S. S., Ed.), Vol. 2. WW 2. New York: Academic Press 1962

Dalen, H., Todd, P. W.: Surface morphology of trypsinized human cells in vitro. Exp. Cell Res. **66**, 353–361 (1971)

David, H.: Zur submikroskopischen Morphologie intrazellulären Gallenkapillaren. Acta anat. (Basel) **47**, 216–224 (1961)

Delorme, P.: Différenciation ultrastructurale des jonctions intercellulaires de l'endothélium des capillaires télencéphaliques chez l'embryon de Poulet. Z. Zellforsch. **133**, 571–582 (1972)

Doolin, P. F., Birge, W. J.: Ultrastructural differentiation of the junctional complex of the avian choroidal epithelium. J. Comp. Neurol. **136**, 253–268 (1969)

Dupuy-Coin, A. M., Bouteille, M.: Developmental pathway of granular and beaded nuclear bodies from nucleoli. J. Ultrastruct. Res. **40**, 55–67 (1972)

Dvorak, M.: Elektronenmikroskopische Untersuchungen an embryonalen Leberzellen. Z. Zellforsch. **62**, 655–666 (1964)

Dvorak, M., Mazanec, K.: Differenzierung der Feinstruktur der Leberzelle in der frühen postnatalen Periode. Z. Zellforsch. **80**, 370–384 (1967)

Eagle, H.: The minimum vitamin requirements of the L and HeLa cells in tissue culture, the production of specific vitamin deficiencies, and their cure. J. exp. Med. **102**, 595–600 (1955)

Eagle, H.: The specific amino acid requirements of a human carcinoma cell (Strain HeLa) in tissue culture. J. exp. Med. **102**, 37–48 (1955)

Eguchi, Y., Hashimoto, Y.: Histological observation of the fetal bovine thyroid. Jap. J. Zootechn. Sci. **30**, 103–108 (1959)

Elias, H., Bengelsdorf, H.: The structure of the liver of Vertebrates. Acta anat. (Basel) **14**, 297–337 (1952)

Escola-Pico, J.: Die Feinstruktur versenkter Ependymozellen innerhalb von gliösen Narbenbereichen. Acta Neuropath. (Berl.) **3**, 137–143 (1963)

Farquhar, M. G., Palade, G. E.: Junctional complexes in various epithelia. J. Cell Biol. **17**, 375–412 (1963)

Fayet, G.: Propriétés des cellules thyroïdiennes de Porc en culture. Régulation de leur organisation en follicule par la thyrotropine in vitro. Thèse Sci. Nat., Marseille 1974

Fayet, G., Lissitzky, S.: Cyclic 3'-5' adenosine monophosphate-mediated follicular reorganization of isolated cells in culture. Febs Lett. II, 185–188 (1970)

Fayet, G., Michel-Béchet, M., Lissitzky, S.: Thyrotrophin-induced aggregation and reorganization into follicles of isolated porcine-thyroid cells in culture. 2. Ultrastructural studies. Europ. J. Biochem. **24**, 100–111 (1971)

Fayet, G., Pacheco, H., Tixier, R.: Sur la réassociation in vitro des cellules isolées de thyroïde de Porc et la biosynthèse de la thyroglobuline. I. Conditions pour l'induction des réassociations cellulaires par la thyréostimuline. Bull. Soc. Chim. biol. **52**, 299–306 (1970)

Fayet, G., Stahl, A., Lissitzky, S.: Microcinématographie du comportement d'une population de cellules thyroïdiennes fraîchement isolées en présence d'hormone thyréotrope. (Agrégation, formation et croissance des follicules, fusion folliculaire, désagrégation, perte de l'architecture et formation d'une monocouche stricte). Film unpublished 1971

Fayet, G., Tixier, R.: Réassociation in vitro de cellules isolées de thyroïde de Porc adulte et biosynthèse d'une protéine apparentée à la thyroglobuline. C. R. Acad. Sci. **265**, 1554–1556 (1967)

Feldman, M.: Dissociation and reaggregation of embryonic cells of Triturus alpestris. J. Embryol. exp. Morph. **3**, 251–255 (1955)

Feldman, J. D., Vazquez, J. J., Kurtz, S. M.: Maturation of the Rat fetal thyroid. J. biophys. biochem. Cytol. **II**, 365–383 (1961)

Florentin, P.: Quelques particularités de l'histogénèse de la glande thyroïde chez les Poissons téléostéens. C. R. Soc. Biol. **109**, 467–469 (1932)

Florentin, P.: La glande thyroïde des Mammifères. Nancy: G. Thomas 1932

Follet, E. A. C., Goldman, R. D.: The occurrence of microvilli during spreading and growth of BHK 21/C 13 fibroblasts. Exp. Cell Res. **59**, 124–136 (1970)

Forte, G. M., Limlomwongse, L., Forte, J. G.: The development of intracellular membranes concomitant with the appearance of HCl secretion in oxyntic cells of the metamorphosing Bullfrog tadpole. J. Cell Sci. **4**, 709–727 (1969)

Franceschini, P., Motta, P.: Fine structure of the Chick embryo liver cell in vivo and in vitro. Acta Morph. Acad. Sci. hungar. **28**, 43–54 (1970)

Fujisawa, H.: The process of reconstruction of histological architecture from dissociated retinal cells. Wilhelm-Roux' Archives **171**, 312–330 (1973)

Fujita, H.: Electron microscopic studies on the thyroid gland of domestic Fowl, with special reference to the mode of secretion and the occurence of a central flagellum in the follicular cell. Z. Zellforsch. **60**, 615–632 (1963)

Fujita, H., Machino, M.: On the follicle formation of the thyroid gland in the Chick embryo. Exp. Cell Res. **25**, 204–206 (1961)

Fujita, H., Murakami, T.: Scanning electron microscopy on the distribution of the minute blood vessels in the thyroid gland of the Dog, Rat and Rhesus Monkey. Arch. Histol. Jap. **36**, 181–188 (1974)

Fujita, H., Tanizawa, Y.: Electron microscopic studies on the development of the thyroid gland of Chick embryo. Z. Anat. Entwickl.-Gesch. **125**, 132–151 (1966)

Gaillard, J. P.: Growth and differentiation of explanted tissues. 4. Culture of thyroid gland from Chick embryos. Int. Rev. Cytol. **2**, 361–367 (1953)

Garber, B. B.: Brain histogenesis in vitro: reconstruction of brain tissue from dissociated cells. In Vitro 8, 167–174 (1972)

Garcia-Bunuel, R., Anton, E., Brandes, D.: The development of lysosomes in the human fetal thyroid in correlation with the onset of functional maturation. Endocrinology **91**, 438–449 (1972)

Garnett, H., Jones, B. M., Kemp, R. B.: Immunofluorescent detection of a myosin type protein at the surface of trypsin-dissociated embryonic Chick cells. Cytobios **7**, 163–169 (1973)

Gerisch, G.: Cell aggregation and differentiation in Dictyostelium. In: Current Topics in Developmental Biology. (Moscona, A. A., Monroy, A., Eds.), p. 157–196. New York: Academic Press 1968

Gierke, v., E.: Drüsen mit innerer Sekretion. Schilddrüse. L. Aschoff's Pathologische Anatomie, 6. Aufl., Bd. 2, p. 906–954. Jena: G. Fischer 1923. Cited by Sugiyama 1971

Giraud, A.: Etude des facteurs d'aggrégation des cellules thyroïdiennes de Porc en culture. Thèse Sci., Marseille 1974

Goebel, H. H., Cravioto, H.: Ultrastructure of human and experimental ependymomas. A comparative study. J. Neuropath. exp. Neurol. **31**, 54–71 (1972)

Goldman, R. D., Follett, E. A. C.: The structure of the major cell processes of isolated BHK 21 fibroblasts. Exp. Cell Res. **57**, 263–276 (1969)

Grosser, O.: Die Entwicklung des Kiemendarmes und des Respirationsapparates. Keibel-Mall's Handbuch der Entwicklungsgeschichte des Menschen. Bd. 2, p. 436–482. Leipzig: S. Hirzel 1911. Cited by Norris 1916, Sugiyama 1971

Hajos, F., Straznicky, I., Mess, B.: The effect of TSH on the ultrastructure of embryonic Chick thyroid. Acta biol. Acad. Sci. hung. **15**, 237–249 (1964)

Hall, A. R., Kaan, H. W.: Anatomical and physiological studies on the thyroid gland of the albino Rat. Anat. Rec. **84**, 221–239 (1942)

Hammar, J. A.: A quelle époque de la vie foetale de l'Homme apparaissent les premiers signes d'une activité endocrine? Etude sur le système endocrine du foetus humain, principalement pendant les deuxième et troisième mois de la gestation au point de vue de la constitution anatomique. Upsala Läk.-Fören. Förh. **30**, 392–480 (1925). Cited by Taki 1959 and Sugiyama 1971

Harris, M.: Cell culture and somatic variation. New York: Holt, Rinehart & Winston 1964

Hayward, A. F.: The fine structure of developing gastric parietal cells in the foetal Rabbit. J. Anat. (Lond.) **101**, 69–81 (1967)

Heimann, P.: Ultrastructure of human thyroid. Acta endocr. (Kbh.) **53**/suppl. 110 (1966)

Helander, H. F.: Ultrastructure and function of gastric parietal cells in the Rat during development. Gastroenterology **56**, 35–52 (1969)

Henkart, P., Humphreys, S., Humphreys, T.: Characterization of Sponge aggregation factor. A unique proteoglycan complex. Biochemistry (Wash.) **12**, 3045–3050 (1973)

Hertwig, O.: Précis d'embryologie de l'Homme et des Vertébrés. p. 249–250. Paris: G. Steinheil 1906

Heyningen, v., H. E.: The initiation of thyroid function in the Mouse. Endocrinology **69**, 720–727 (1961)

Hilfer, S. R.: Follicle formation in the embryonic Chick thyroid. I. Early morphogenesis. J. Morph. **115**, 135–152 (1964)

Hilfer, S. R.: Cellular interactions in the genesis and maintenance of thyroid characteristics. In: Epithelial-mesenchymal interactions, (Fleischmajer R. & Billingham R. E., Eds.), p. 177–199. Baltimore: Williams and Wilkins Cy 1968

Hilfer, S. R., Hilfer, E. K.: Effects of dissociating agents on the fine structure of embryonic Chick thyroid cells. J. Morph. **119**, 217–231 (1966)

Hilfer, S. R., Hilfer, E. K., Iszard, L. B.: The relationship between cytoplasmic organization and the epithelio-mesodermal interactions in the embryonic Chick thyroid. J. Morph. **123**, 199–212 (1967)

Hilfer, S. R., Iszard, L. B., Hilfer, E. K.: Follicle formation in the embryonic Chick thyroid. II. Reorganization after dissociation. Z. Zellforsch. **92**, 256–269 (1968)

Hirano, A., Zimmerman, H. M.: Some new cytological observations of the normal Rat ependymal cells. Anat. Rec. **158**, 293–302 (1967)

His, W.: Anatomie menschlicher Embryonen. 3. p. 60–72. Leipzig: F. C. W. Vogel 1885. Cited by Minot 1894 and Norris 1916

Hoar, W. H.: The thyroid gland of the atlantic Salmon. J. Morph. **65**, 257–295 (1939)

Hodges, G. M., Livingston, D. C., Franks, L. M.: The localization of trypsin in cultured mammalian cells. J. Cell Sci. **12**, 887–902 (1973)

Hopkins, M. L.: Development of the thyroid gland in the Chick embryo. J. Morph. **58**, 585–613 (1935)

Horcika, J.: Beiträge zur Entwicklungs- und Wachstumsgeschichte der Schilddrüse. Prag. Z. Heilk. I, 1880. Cited by Norris 1916

Hosick, H. L., Strohman, R. C.: Changes in ribosome-polyribosome balance in Chick muscle cells during tissue dissociation, development in culture and exposure to simplified culture medium. J. cell Physiol. **77**, 145–156 (1971)

Hourdry, J.: Remaniements ultrastructuraux de l'épithélium intestinal chez la larva d'un Amphibien Anoure en métamorphose. II. Phénomènes histogénétiques. Z. Zellforsch. **101**, 555–567 (1969)

Hugon, J. S., Borgers, M.: Ultrastructural differentiation and enzymatic localization of phosphatases in the developing duodenal epithelium of the Mouse. I. The foetal Mouse. Histochemie **19**, 13–30 (1969)

Humphreys, T.: Cell surface components participating in aggregation: evidence for a new cell particulate. Exp. Cell Res. **40**, 539–543 (1965)

Hürthle, K.: Beiträge zur Kenntnis des Sekretionsvorgangs in der Schilddrüse. Pflüger's Arch. ges. Physiol. **20**, 267–270 (1894). Cited by Norris 1916

Ishikawa, K.: Electron microscopic studies on the thyroid gland of the Rat in embryonic life. Okajimas Folia anat. jap. **41**, 295–311 (1965)

Iwig, M., Weber, E., Friedrich, E., Glaesser, D.: Isolation and identification of aggregation promoting substances from the bovine eye lens. Febs Lett. **30**, 210–214 (1973)

Jones, B. M., Kemp, R. B., Aggregation and electrophoretic mobility studies on dissociated cells. II. Effects of ADP and ATP. Exp. Cell Res. **63**, 301–308 (1970)

Jokelainen, P.: An electron microscope study of the early development of the Rat metanephric nephron. Acta Anat. (Basel) 52/suppl. **47**, 1–101 (1963)

Jones, A. L.: Preliminary observations on the developing biliary system in Chick embryos. Ann. N. Y. Acad. Sci. III, 157–160 (1963)

Jost, A.: Sur le développement de la thyroïde chez le foetus de Lapin décapité. Arch. Anat. micr. Morph. exp. **42**, 168–183 (1953)

Junqueira, L. C.: Action in vitro of thyrotrophic hormone and iodine on thyroid cells. Endocrinology **40**, 286–291 (1947)

Kalderon, A. E., Wittner, M.: Histochemical studies of thyroid cells in long-term tissue culture. Endocrinology **80**, 797–807 (1967)

Kalnins, V. I., Porter, K. R.: Centriole replication during ciliogenesis in the Chick tracheal epithelium. Z. Zellforsch. **100**, 1–30 (1969)

Karrer, H. E., Cox, J.: Electron microscope observations on Chick embryo liver: glycogen, bile canaliculi, inclusions bodies and hematopoiesis. J. Ultrastruct. Res. **5**, 116–141 (1961)

Kelly, D. E., Luft, J. H.: Fine structure, development and classification of desmosomes and related attachment mechanisms. 6th Intern. Congr. for Electron Microscopy (Uyeda, R., Ed.), p. 401–402. Tokyo: Maruzen Co. 1966

Kerkof, P. R., Long, P. J.: Chaikoff, I. L.: In vitro effects of thyrotropic hormone. I. On the pattern of organization of monolayer cultures of isolated Sheep thyroid gland cells. Endocrinology **74**, 170–179 (1964)

Khairallah, L. H., Clark, N. B.: Ultrastructure and histochemistry of the ultimobranchial body of fresh-water Turtles. Z. Zellforsch. **113**, 311–321 (1971)

Knake, E., Riedel, B.: Organstruktur und Zellfunktion in explantiertem und später retransplantiertem Schilddrüsengewebe. Z. Zellforsch. **52**, 408–426 (1960)

Koga, A.: Morphogenesis of intrahepatic bile ducts of the human fetus. Light and electron microscopic study. Z. Anat. Entwickl.-Gesch. **135**, 156–184 (1971)

Kojima, M.: Tissue culture studies on the differentiation and function of the thyroid gland. Bull. Tokyo med. dent. Univ. **7**, 37–44 (1960)

Kölliker, A.: Grundriß der Entwicklungsgeschichte des Menschen und der höheren Tiere. p. 367–369. Leipzig: W. Engelmann 1884

Koneff, A. A., Nichols, C. W., Wolff, J., Chaikoff, I. L.: The fetal bovine thyroid: morphogenesis as related to iodine accumulation. Endocrinology **45**, 242–249 (1949)

Kraentzel, F.: Contribution à l'étude de la Lamproie fluviatile, Lampetra (Petromyzon) fluviatilis, L. 1. La transformation de l'endostyle en glande thyroïde. 2. La formation de l'oesophage de la Lamproie. Arch. Biol. (Liège) **44**, 469–517 (1933)

Kraicziczek, M.: Histogenese und Funktionszustand der embryonalen Hühnerthyreoidea. Z. Zellforsch. **43**, 421–458 (1956)

Krawczyk, W. S., Wilgram, G. F.: Hemidesmosome and desmosome morphogenesis during epidermal wound healing. J. Ultrastruct. Res. **45**, 93–101 (1973)

Kuroda, Y.: Inhibition by cyclic AMP and dibutyryl cyclic AMP of aggregation of embryonic Quail liver cells in culture. Exp. Cell Res. **84**, 303–310 (1974)

Laguesse, E.: Trois leçons sur les glandes à sécrétion interne en général, et en particulier sur la glande endocrine du pancréas. Echo méd. Nord, 21–23 (1925)

Lambiotte, M., Vorbrodt, A., Benedetti, E. L.: Apparition de canalicules biliaires dans le foie foetal de Rat en culture cellulaire sous l'influence de glycocorticoïdes. C. R. Acad. Sci. **275** — Sér. D, 2539–2542 (1972)

Langendorff, O.: Beiträge zur Kenntnis der Schilddrüse. Arch. Physiol. Leipzig, suppl., 218–242 (1889). Cited by Laguesse 1925, Sugiyama 1941, Florentin 1932

Leach, W. J.: The endostyle and thyroid gland of the brook Lamprey, Ichthyomyzon fossor. J. Morph. **65**, 549–605 (1939)

Lennep, v., E. W.: Ultrastructural differentiation of the intestinal epithelium in the Bandicoot Perameles nasuka. Z. Zellforsch. **62**, 485–494 (1964)

Lietz, H., Wöhler, J., Pomp, H.: Zur Entwicklung und Ultrastruktur der embryonalen Schilddrüse des Menschen. Z. Zellforsch. **113**, 94–110 (1971)

Lilien, J. E., Moscona, A. A.: Cell aggregation: its enhancement by a supernatant from cultures of homologous cells. Science **157**, 70–72 (1967)

Lissitzky, S., Fayet, G., Verrier, B., Hennen, G., Jaquet, P.: Thyroid-stimulating hormone binding to cultured thyroid cells. Febs Lett. **29**, 20–24 (1973)

Loeschke, E.: Morphologische Untersuchungen über den Bau der normalen und pathologischen Schilddrüse. Beitr. path. Anat. **98**, 521–544 (1937). Cited by Taki 1959 and Sugiyama 1971

Loewenstein, W. R.: On the genesis of cellular communication. Develop. Biol. **15**, 503–520 (1967)

Loewenstein, W. R.: Membrane junctions in growth and differentiation. Fed. Proc. **32**, 60–64 (1973)

Lucien, M., Parisot, J., Richard, G.: La thyroïde, p. 92–95. Paris: G. Doin 1925

Luse, S. A.: Electron microscopic studies of brain tumors. Neurology (Minneap.) **10**, 881–905 (1960)

Lustig, A.: Contribution à la connaissance de l'histogénèse de la glande thyroïde. Arch. ital. Biol. **15**, 291–295 (1891). Cited by Norris 1916, Florentin 1932

Macario, C.: Contribution à l'étude de la thyroïde embryonnaire des Vertébrés Amniotes. Thèse Méd., Bordeaux: Delmas 1954

Mallette, J. M., Anthony, A.: Growth in culture of trypsin dissociated thyroid cells from adult Rats. Exp. Cell Res. **41**, 642–651 (1966)

Maraud, R., Stoll, R.: Sur la fonction thyroïdienne chez l'embryon des Vertébrés Amniotes. Biol. Méd. (Paris) L, 313–352 (1961)

Marshall, A. M.: Vertebrate embryology. p. 285–286. New-York: G. P. Putnam's Sons 1893. Cited by Norris 1916, Bradway 1929

Martinez-Martinez, P., Daems, W. T.: Les phases précoces de la formation des cils et le problème de l'origine du corpuscule basal. Z. Zellforsch. **87**, 46–68 (1968)

Martinez-Palomo, A.: The surface coats of animal cells. Int. Rev. Cytol. **29**, 29–75 (1970)

Mason, J. W., Rasmussen, H. Dibella, F.: 3'–5' AMP and Ca^{2+} in slime mold aggregation. Exp. Cell Res. **67**, 156–160 (1971)

Mauchamp, J., Fayet, G.: Three dimensional reorganization of thyroid cells in culture and iodide metabolism. VIth Ann. Meet. Europ. Thyroid Assoc., Prague 1974. Abstract 17

Michel-Bechet, M., Cau, P., Fayet, G.: Etude ultrastructurale de la morphogénèse du follicule thyroïdien: réorganisation des cellules thyroïdiennes de Porc en culture. C. R. Acad. Sci. Paris 277 Série D, 1029–1032 (1973)

Michel-Bechet, M., Cotte, G., Codaccioni, J. L., Athouel-Haon, A. M.: Ultrastructure thyroïdienne et perturbations biochimiques de l'hormonogénèse. Acta Anat. (Basel) **73**, 389–409 (1969)

Michel-Bechet, M., Cotte, G., Haon, A. M.: Aspect ultrastructural microfolliculaire de formations épithéliales compactes dans des thyroïdes humaines pathologiques. Bull. Ass. Anat. (Nancy) **142**, 1238–1246 (1968)

Millonig, G., Giudice, G.: Electron microscopic study of the reaggregation of cells dissociated from sea Urchin embryos. Develop. Biol. **15**, 91–101 (1967)

Minot, C. S.: Lehrbuch der Entwicklungsgeschichte des Menschen, p. 774–779. Leipzig: Von Veitland 1894

Moscona, A. A.: Studies on cell aggregation: demonstration of materials with selective cell-binding activity. Proc. nat. Acad. Sci. (Wash.) **49**, 742–747 (1963)

Moscona, A. A.: Recombination of dissociated cells and the development of cell aggregates. In: Cells and Tissues in culture (Wilmer, E. N., Ed.), p. 489–529. London: Academic Press 1966

Mugnaini, E., Harboe, S. B., The liver of Myxine glutinosa: a true tubular gland. Z. Zellforsch. **78**, 341–369 (1967)

Müller, W.: Über die Entwicklung der Schilddrüse. Jena Z. Med. Naturw. **6**, 428 (1871). Cited by Norris 1916, Sugiyama 1941

Muller, W. E. G., Zahn, R. K.: Isolation and characterization of a species-specific aggregation factor in Sponges. Exp. Cell Res. **10**, 95–104 (1973)

Neve, P.: Ultrastructure of the thyroid in de Quervain's subacute granulomatous thyroiditis. Virchows Arch. path. Anat., Abt. A 35, 87 (1970)

Neve, P., Dumont, J. E.: Time sequence of ultrastructural changes in the stimulated Dog thyroid. Z. Zellforsch. **103**, 61–74 (1970)

Neve, P., Rodesch, F. R., Dumont, J. E.: Electron microscopy of isolated sheep thyroid cells. Exp. Cell Res. **51**, 68–78 (1968)

Nomura, Y.: On the submicroscopic morphogenesis of parietal cells in the gastric gland of the human fetus. Z. Anat. Entwickl.-Gesch. **125**, 316–356 (1966)

Nonaka, T.: Experimental embryological studies on the early development of the thyroid gland in Amphibia. Okajimas Folia anat. jap. **28**, 489–506 (1956)

Nonaka, T., Watanabe, T., Sato, S., Shimada, T.: On the differentiation of primordial thyroid of amphibian embryo and its I^{131} uptake rate. Okajimas Folia anat. jap. **32**, 319–327 (1959)

Norris, E. H.: The morphogenesis of the follicles in the human thyroid gland. Amer. J. Anat. **20**, 3 411–448 (1916)

Novikoff, A. B., Noe, E. F.: Observations on fragmented Rat liver canaliculi and the problems of intracellular bile canaliculi and Golgi apparatus. J. Morph. **96**, 189–221 (1955)

Ono, K.: The fine structural localization of alkaline phosphatase activity of intestinal microvilli in the developing Chick embryo. Acta Anat. (Basel) **86**, 71–82 (1973)

Osathanondh, V., Potter, E. L.: Development of human kidney as shown by microdissection. IV. Development of tubular portions of nephrons. Arch. Path. **82**, 391–402 (1966)

Overton, J.: Desmosome development in normal and reassociating cells in early Chick blastoderm. Develop. Biol. **4**, 532–548 (1962)

Overton, J.: The fate of desmosomes in trypsinized tissue. J. exp. Zool. **168**, 203–214 (1968)

Overton, J.: Experimental manipulation of desmosome formation. J. Cell Biol. **56**, 636–646 (1973)

Overton, J., Culver, N.: Desmosomes and their components after cell dissociation and reaggregation in the presence of cytochalasin B. J. exp. Zool. **185**, 341–356 (1973)

Peremeschko: Ein Beitrag zum Bau der Schilddrüse. Z. wiss. Zool. **17**, (1867). Cited by Norris 1916, Sugiyama 1941

Pessac, B., Alliot, F., Girouard, A.: Etude in vitro des mécanismes de l'adhésion intercellulaire chez l'embryon de Poulet: effect du sérum. C. R. Acad. Sci. **276**, 3465–3468 (1973)

Pessac, B., Defendi, V.: Evidence for distinct aggregation factors and receptors in cells. Nature New Biol. (Lond.) **238**, 13–15 (1972)

Peters, V. B., Kelly, G. W., Dembitzer, H. M.: Cytologic changes in fetal and neonatal hepatic cells of the Mouse. Ann. N. Y. Acad. Sci. 111, 87–103 (1963)

Petrovic, A., Porte, A.: Sur la formation en culture organotypique de lacunes intercellulaires dans la thyroïde d'embryon de Poulet de six jours et demi. Etude sous l'influence de la thyréostimuline. Etude au microscope électronique. C. R. Soc. Biol. **155**, 1848–1855 (1961)

Phelps, C. H.: The development of glio-vascular relationship in the Rat spinal cord. An electron microscopic study. Z. Zellforsch. **128**, 555–563 (1972)

Pictet, R. L., Clark, W. R., Williams, R. H., Rutter, W. J.: An ultrastructural analysis of the developing embryonic pancreas. Develop. Biol. **29**, 436–467 (1972)

Poon, T. P., Hirano, A., Zimmerman, H. M.: Electron microscopic atlas of brain tumors. New York: Grune & Stratton Inc. 1971

Prenant, A., Bouin, P., Maillard, L.: Traité d'Histologie. Tome II, p. 970–977. Paris: Masson et Cie 1911

Pulaski, A.: Vergleichende histologische Untersuchungen an foetalen Schilddrüsen aus Hamburg und Bern. Frankfurt Z. Path. **38**, 29–63 (1929). Cited by Taki 1959, Sugiyama 1971

Rambourg, A.: Morphological and histochemical aspects of glycoproteins at the surface of animal cells. Intern. Rev. Cytol. **31**, 57–114 (1970)

Remak, R.: Untersuchungen über die Entwicklung der Wirbeltiere. p. 122–123. Berlin: J. Reimer 1855. Cited by Norris 1916. Venzke 1949

Renaud, F. L., Swift, H.: The development of basal bodies and flagella in Allomyces arbusculus. J. Cell Biol. **23**, 339–354 (1964)

Richmond, J. E., Glaeser, R. M., Todd, P.: Protein synthesis in aggregation of embryonic cells. Exp. Cell Res. **52**, 43–58 (1968)

Robertis, de, E.: Proteolytic enzyme activity of colloid extracted from single follicles of the Rat thyroid. Anat. Rec. **80**, 219–231 (1941)

Robertson, A., Drage, D. J., Cohen, M. H.: Control of aggregation in Dictyostelium discoideum by an external periodic pulse of cyclic adenosine monophosphate. Science **175**, 333–335 (1972)

Rodesch, F. R., Neve, P., Dumont, J. E.: Phagocytosis of latex beads by isolated thyroid cells. Exp. Cell Res. **60**, 354–360 (1970)

Röhlich, P.: Formation of the brush border by fusion of vesicles. 5th Intern. Congr. Electron Micr. Philadelphia (Breese S. S., Ed.), vol. 2, LL5. New York: Academic Press 1962

Roques, M., Torresani, J., Michel-Bechet, M., Jost, A., Lissitzky, S.: Relationship between thyroglobulin synthesis, iodine metabolism, and histogenesis in the developing Rabbit fetal thyroid gland. Gen. comp. Endocr. 19, 457–472 (1972)

Rose, G. G.: Atlas of vertebrate cells in tissue culture. London: Academic Press 1970

Roseman, S.: The synthesis of complex carbohydrates by multiglycosyltransferase systems and their potential function in intercellular adhesion. Chem. Phys. Lip. 5, 270–297 (1970)

Roth, S.: Studies on intercellular adhesive selectivity. Develop. Biol. 18, 602–631 (1968)

Roth, S.: A molecular model for cell interactions. Quart. Rev. Biol. 48, 541–563 (1973)

Saxen, L., Wartiovaara, J.: Cell contact and cell adhesion during tissue organization. Intern. J. Cancer 1, 271–290 (1966)

Schreckenberg, G.: The embryonic development of the thyroid gland in the Frog, Hyla brunnea. Growth 20, 295–313 (1956)

Sedar, A. W.: Electron microscopy of the oxyntic cell in the gastric gland of the Bullfrog, Rana catesbeiana. II. The acid-secreting gastric mucosa. J. biophys. biochem. Cytol. 10, 47–57 (1961)

Sedar, A. W.: Electron microscopic demonstration of polysaccharides associated with acid secreting cells of the stomach after inert dehydration. J. Ultrastruct. Res. 28, 112–124 (1969a)

Sedar, A. W.: Uptake of peroxidase into the smooth surfaced tubular system of the gastric acid-secreting cell. J. Cell Biol. 43, 179–184 (1969b)

Shaw-Dunn, J.: The fine structure of the absorptive epithelial cells of the developing small intestine of the Rat. J. Anat. (Lond.) 101, 57–68 (1967)

Sheffield, J. B., Moscona, A. A.: Early stages in the reaggregation of embryonic Chick neural retina cells. Exp. Cell Res. 57, 462–466 (1969)

Sheffield, J. B., Moscona, A. A.: Electron microscopic analysis of aggregation of embryonic cells: the structure and differentiation of aggregates of neural retina cells. Develop. Biol. 23, 36–61 (1970)

Shelburne, J. D., Arstila, A. U., Trump, B. F.: Studies on cellular autophagocytosis: cyclic AMP- und dibutyryl cyclic AMP-stimulated autophagy in Rat liver. Amer. J. Path. 72, 521–540 (1973)

Shepard, T. H.: Onset of function in the human fetal thyroid: biochemical and radioautographic studies from organ culture. J. clin. Endocr. 27, 945–958 (1967)

Shepard, T. H.: Development of the human fetal thyroid. Gen. comp. Endocr. 10, 174–181 (1968)

Shimazaki, M., Shiozaki, A., Hiramine, C., Mori, T., Katsu, N., Otsui, A.: An electron microscopic study on cytotoxic susceptibility of cultured human thyroid epithelial cells. Wakayama Med. Reports II, 143–152 (1967)

Sigot, M.: Dissociation des cellules et réassociation in vitro. In: Les cultures organotypiques (Thomas, J. A., Ed.), p. 255–282. Paris: Masson & Cie 1965

Simar, L. J.: Ultrastructure et constitution des corps nucléaires dans les plasmocytes. Z. Zellforsch. 99, 235–251 (1969)

Simpson, B. T.: Growth centers of the benign blastoma with special reference to thyroid and prostatic adenomata. J. med. Res. 22, 269–284 (1912)

Smeds, S.: The proteins of the thyroid colloid. A study of single rat thyroid follicles by microgel electrophoresis. Thesis, Göteborg 1972

Smith, J. W., Christie, K. N., Frame, J.: Desmosomes, cilia and acanthosomes associated with keratocytes. J. Anat. (Lond.) 105, 383–392 (1969)

Sobel, H., Leurer, H.: Effects of thyrotropin and thiouracil on embryonic Chick thyroid in vitro. Experientia (Basel) 14, 213–214 (1958)

Sorokin, S.: Centrioles and the formation of rudimentary cilia by fibroblasts and smooth muscle cells. J. Cell Biol. 15, 363–377 (1962)

Spooner, B. S.: The expression of differentiation by Chick embryo thyroid in cell culture. I. Functional and fine structural stability in mass and clonal culture. J. cell Physiol. 75, 33–48 (1970)

Spooner, B. S., Ash, J. F., Wrenn, J. T., Frater, R. B., Wessels, N. K.: Heavy meromyosin binding to microfilaments involved in cell and morphogenetic movements. Tissue & Cell 5, 37–46 (1973)

Starre van der-Molen van der, L. G., Priester de, W.: Brush-border formation in the midgut of an Insect, Calliphora erythrocephala Meigen. The formation of microvilli in the midgut during embryonic development. Z. Zellforsch. **125**, 295–305 (1972)

Stefko, W. H.: Beiträge zur Kenntnis Konstitutions-anatomischer Besonderheit der Organe. (vom Standpunkte der postnatalen Entwicklung). Z. Konstit.-Lehre **18**, 287–310 (1934). Cited by Taki 1959, Sugiyama 1971

Steinberg, M. S.: "E. C. M.": its nature, origin and function in cell aggregation. Exp. Cell Res. **30**, 257–279 (1963)

Steinberg, M. S., Armstrong, P. B., Granger, R. E.: On the recovery of adhesiveness by trypsin-dissociated cells. J. Membrane Biol. **13**, 97–128 (1973)

Stern, S. M.: Experimental studies on the organization of the preimplantation Mouse embryo. II. Reaggregation of disaggregated embryos. J. Embryol. exp. Morph. **28**, 255–261 (1972)

Stieda, L.: Untersuchungen über die Entwicklung der Glandula Thymus, Glandula thyroidea und Glandula carotica. Leipzig: 1881. Cited by Norris 1916, Florentin 1932

Stoll, R., Maraud, R., Capot, L.: Sur l'histophysiologie de la thyroïde de l'embryon de Poulet. C. R. Assoc. Anat. **81**, 785–806 (1953)

Streiff, J. J.: Über die Form der Schilddrüsen-Follikel des Menschen. Arch. mikr. Anat. **48**, 579–586 (1897). Cited by Norris 1916, Taki 1959, and Sugiyama 1971

Strum, J. M., Wicken, J., Stanbury, J. R., Karnovsky, M. J.: Appearance and function of endogenous peroxidase in fetal Rat thyroid. J. Cell Biol. **51**, 162–175 (1971)

Stubblefield, E., Brinkley, B. R.: Architecture and function of the mammalian centriole: ciliogenesis. In: Formation and fate of cells organelles (Brehme Warren, K., Ed.), p. 200–203. London: Academic Press 1967

Sugiyama, S.: The embryonic development of the thyroid gland in the albino Rat and the Mouse with special emphasis on its histogenesis. Okajimas Folia anat. jap. **20**, 465–506 (1941)

Sugiyama, S.: The embryology of the human thyroid gland including ultimobranchial body and others related. Ergebn. Anat. Entwickl.-Gesch. 44/2 (1971)

Suzuki, S., Kondo, Y.: Thyroidal morphogenesis and biosynthesis of thyroglobulin before and after metamorphosis in the Lamprey, Lampetra reissneri. Gen. comp. Endocr. **21**, 451–460 (1973)

Takashima, R., Hara, S.: Über die Entwicklung der Schilddrüse beim Japaner. Z. Anat. Entwickl.-Gesch. **102**, 409–423 (1934)

Taki, A.: Histological studies of the prenatal development of the human thyroid gland. Okajimas Folia anat. jap. **32**, 65–85 (1959)

Timourian, H., Clothier, G., Watchmaker, G.: Reaggregation of sea Urchin blastula cells. I. Intrinsic differences in the blastula cells. Develop. Biol. **31**, 252–263 (1973)

Tixier-Vidal, A.: Etude histophysiologique des relations hypophyse et thyroïde chez l'embryon de Poulet. Arch. Anat. micr. Morph. exp. 47/suppl., 235–340 (1958)

Tixier-Vidal, A., Picart, R., Rappaport, L., Nunez, J.: Ultrastructure et autoradiographie de cellules thyroïdiennes isolées, incubées en présence de [125]I. J. Ultrastruct. Res. **28**, 78–101 (1969)

Togari, C., Sugiyama, S., Sawasaki, Y.: On the prenatal histogenesis of the thyroid gland of the Rabbit with special emphasis on its histometrical measurements. Anat. Rec. **114**, 213–222 (1952)

Tonegawa, Y.: Isolation and characterization of a particulate cell-aggregation factor from sea Urchin embryos. Develop. Growth. Different. **14**, 337–352 (1973)

Tong, W., Kerkof, P., Chaikoff, I. L.: Iodine metabolism of dispersed thyroid cells obtained by trypsinisation of Sheep thyroid glands. Biochim. Biophys. Acta **60**, 1–19 (1962)

Tourneux, F., Verdun, P.: Sur les premiers développements de la thyroïde, du thymus et des glandes parathyroïdiennes chez l'Homme. J. Anat. Physiol. (Paris) **33**, 305–325 (1893)

Tyler, A.: An auto-antibody concept of cell structure in growth. Growth 10/Suppl., 7–19 (1947). Cited by Weiss, P. 1958, Weiss, L. 1960, Curtiss 1962

Vague, J., Alland, A., Michel-Bechet, M., Jean, R.: Les nodules thyroïdiens actifs. In: La Thyroïde, vol. II (Zara, M., Ed.), p. 279–328. Paris: Expansion Scientifique Française 1972

Vague, J., Michel-Bechet, M., Cotte, G., Lieutaud, R., Alland, A., Simonin, R.: Preliminary observations on optical and electron microscopical pathology of autonomous secreting nodules of thyroid. In: Thyroid neoplasias, p. 345–362. London: Academic Press 1968

Venzke, W. G.: Morphogenesis of the thyroid glands of Chicken embryos. Amer. J. et. Res. **10**, 272–281 (1949)

Vetter, S. M. R., Gibley, J. C. W.: Morphogenesis and histochemistry of the developing Mouse kidney. J. Morph. **120**, 135–156 (1966)

Vial, J. D., Orrego, H.: Electron microscope observations on the fine structure of parietal cells. J. biophys. biochem. Cytol. **7**, 367–372 (1960)

Voikevich, A. A., Zenzerov, V. S.: Intracellular formation of thyroid follicles. Tsitologiya **10**, 945–952 (1968)

Vollrath, L.: Über die Mikrovillibildung im fetalen Rattendünndarm. Z. Zellforsch. **114**, 546–556 (1971)

Volpe, R., Row, V. V., Ezrin, C.: Circulating viral and thyroid antibodies in subacute thyroiditis. J. Clin. Endocr. **27**, 1275 (1967).

Vos de, R., Wolf-Peeters de, C., Desmet, V.: A morphologic and histochemical study of biliary atresia in Lamprey liver. Z. Zellforsch. **136**, 85–96 (1973)

Wartiovaara, J.: Studies on kidney tubulogenesis. V. Electron microscopy of basement membrane formation in vitro. Ann. Med. exp. Fenn. **44**, 140–150 (1966a)

Wartiovaara, J.: Cell contacts in relation to cytodifferentiation in metanephrogenic mesenchyme in vitro. Ann. Med. exp. Fenn. **44**, 469–503 (1966b)

Weil, A.: Die innere Sekretion, 2. Aufl., S. 1–146. Berlin: Springer 1922. Cited by Sugiyama 1971

Weiss, L.: Studies on cellular adhesion in tissue culture. XII A. Some effects of prostaglandins and cyclic nucleotides. Exp. Cell Res. **81**, 57–62 (1973)

Weiss, P.: Cell contact. Int. Rev. Cytol. **7**, 391–423 (1958)

Weissman, G., Dingle, J.: Release of lysosomal protease by ultraviolet irridiation and inhibition by hydrocortisone. Exp. Cell Res. **25**, 207 (1961)

Welsch, U.: Die Entwicklung der C-Zellen und des Follikel-Epithels der Säugerschilddrüse. Ergebn. Anat. Entwickl.-Gesch. **46**/2 (1972)

Wetzel, B. K., Wollman, S. H.: Fine structure of a second kind of thyroid follicle in the C_3H Mouse. Endocrinology **84**, 563–578 (1969)

Wheatley, D. N.: Cilia and centrioles of the Rat adrenal cortex. J. Anat. (Lond.) **101**, 223–237 (1967)

Wilson, H. V.: On some phenomena of coalescence and regeneration in Sponges. J. exp. Zool. **5**, 245–258 (1907)

Wilson, H. V.: On the behavior of the dissociated cells in Hydroids, Alcyonaria and Asterias. J. exp. Zool. **II**, 281–338 (1911)

Wilson, J. W., Groat, C. S., Leduc, E. H.: Histogenesis of the liver. Ann. N. Y. Acad. Sci. **III**, 8–24 (1963)

Winzler, R. J.: Carbohydrates in cell surfaces. Int. Rev. Cytol. **29**, 77–125 (1970)

Wolfler, A.: Über die Entwicklung und den Bau des Kropfes. Langenbecks Arch. klin. Chir. **29**, 1–97 (1883). Cited by Minot 1894, Norris 1916 Sugiyama 1971

Wolf-Peeters, de, C., Vos, de, R., Desmet, V.: Electron microscopy and histochemistry of canalicular differentiation in fetal and neonatal Rat liver. Tissue Cell **4**, 379–388 (1972)

Wood, R. L.: An electron microscope study of developing bile canaliculi in the Rat. Anat. Rec. **151**, 507–530 (1965)

Yalciner, S., Friedell, G. H.: Cilia in the epithelium of the urinary bladder during experimental carciogenesis. J. nat. Cancer Inst. **51**, 501–505 (1973)

Yatvin, M. G., Wannemacher, P. W., Brown, N. V.: Effects of cortisone on thyroid protein metabolism in euthyroid and thiouracil-treated Rats. Endocrinology **79**, 1079–1086 (1966)

Young, B. A.: Intercellular channels in the canine and porcine thyroid gland. J. A. nat. (Lond.) **100**, 895–898 (1966)

Zamboni, L.: Electron microscopic studies of blood embryogenesis in Humans. I. The ultrastructure of the fetal liver. J. Ultrastruct. Res. **12**, 509–524 (1965)

Zimmerman, K. W.: Beiträge zur Kenntnis einiger Drüsen und Epithelien. Arch. mikr. Anat. **52**, 552–706 (1898)

Subject Index

Advances in Anatomy, Embryology and Cell Biology
Ergebnisse der Anatomie und Entwicklungsgeschichte
Revues d'anatomie et de morphologie expérimentale

Springer-Verlag Berlin Heidelberg New York

This journal publishes reviews and critical articles covering the entire field of normal anatomy (cytology, histology, cyto- and histochemistry, electron microscopy, macroscopy, experimental morphology and embryology and comparative anatomy). Papers dealing with anthropology and clinical morphology will also be accepted with the aim of encouraging co-operation between anatomy and related disciplines.

Papers, which may be in English, French or German, are normally commissioned, but original papers and communications may be submitted and will be considered so long as they deal with a subject comprehensively and meet the requirements of the "Ergebnisse".

For speed of publication and breadth of distribution, this journal appears in single issues which can be purchased separately; 6 issues constitute one volume.

It is a fundamental condition that submitted manuscripts have not been, and will not simultaneously be submitted or published elsewhere. With the acceptance of a manuscript for publication, the publishers acquire full and exclusive copyright for all languages and countries.

25 copies of each paper are supplied free of charge.

Die Ergebnisse dienen der Veröffentlichung zusammenfassender und kritischer Artikel aus dem Gesamtgebiet der normalen Anatomie (Cytologie, Histologie, Cyto- und Histochemie, Elektronenmikroskopie, Makroskopie, experimentelle Morphologie und Embryologie und vergleichende Anatomie). Aufgenommen werden ferner Arbeiten anthropologischen und morphologisch-klinischen Inhaltes, mit dem Ziel, die Zusammenarbeit zwischen Anatomie und Nachbardisziplinen zu fördern.

Zur Veröffentlichung gelangen in erster Linie angeforderte Manuskripte, jedoch werden auch eingesandte Arbeiten und Originalmitteilungen berücksichtigt, sofern sie ein Gebiet umfassend abhandeln und den Anforderungen der ,,Ergebnisse" genügen. Die Veröffentlichungen erfolgen in englischer, deutscher und französischer Sprache.

Die Arbeiten erscheinen im Interesse einer raschen Veröffentlichung und einer weiten Verbreitung als einzeln berechnete Hefte; je 6 Hefte bilden einen Band.

Grundsätzlich dürfen nur Arbeiten eingesandt werden, die nicht gleichzeitig an anderer Stelle zur Veröffentlichung eingereicht oder bereits veröffentlicht worden sind. Der Autor verpflichtet sich, seinen Beitrag auch nachträglich nicht an anderer Stelle zu publizieren.

Die Mitarbeiter erhalten von ihren Arbeiten zusammen 25 Freiexemplare.

Les résultats publient des sommaires et des articles critiques concernant l'ensemble du domaine de l'anatomie normale (cytologie, histologie, cyto- et histochimie, microscopie électronique, macroscopie, morphologie expérimentale, embryologie et anatomie comparée. Seront publiés en outre les articles traitant de l'anthropologie et de la morphologie clinique, en vue d'encourager la collaboration entre l'anatomie et les disciplines voisines.

Seront publiés en priorité les articles expressément demandés, nous tiendrons toutefois compte des articles qui nous seront envoyés dans la mesure où ils traitent d'un sujet dans son ensemble et correspondent aux standards des «Ergebnisse». Les publications seront faites en langues anglaise, allemande et française.

Dans l'intérêt d'une publication rapide et d'une large diffusion les travaux publiés paraitront dans des cahiers individuels, diffusés séparément: 6 cahiers forment un volume.

En principe, seuls les manuscrits qui n'ont encore été publiés ni dans le pays d'origine ni à l'étranger peuvent nous être soumis. L'auteur s'engage en outre à ne pas les publier ailleurs ultérieurement.

Les auteurs recevront 25 exemplaires gratuits de leur publication.

Manuscripts should be addressed to/Envoyer les manuscrits à/Manuskripte sind zu senden an:

Prof. Dr. A. BRODAL, Universitetet i Oslo, Anatomisk Institutt, Karl Johans Gate 47 (Domus Media), Oslo 1/Norwegen

Prof. W. HILD, Department of Anatomy. The University of Texas Medical Branch, Galveston, Texas 77550 (USA)

Prof. Dr. J. van LIMBORGH, Universiteit van Amsterdam, Anatomisch-Embryologisch Laboratorium, Mauritskade 61, Amsterdam-O/Holland

Prof. Dr. R. ORTMANN, Anatomisches Institut der Universität, Lindenburg, D-5000 Köln-Lindenthal

Prof. Dr. T. H. SCHIEBLER, Anatomisches Institut der Universität, Koellikerstraße 6, D-8700 Würzburg

Prof. Dr. G. TÖNDURY, Direktion der Anatomie, Gloriastraße 19, CH-8006 Zürich/Schweiz

Prof. Dr. E. WOLFF, Collège de France, Laboratoire d'Embryologie Expérimentale, 49 bis Avenue de la belle Gabrielle, Nogent-sur-Marne 94/France